PREFACE
TO THE FOURTH EDITION

FOLLOWING the successful development of immunological techniques recently, this edition includes more than fifty new sections, including many hormone estimations. Other sections have been extensively revised and rewritten.

Where relevant, the method of calculation to produce the metric system of units, known as S.I. units (*Système International d'Unités*), has been included, following the recommendation of the Royal Society in 1969; unfortunately those substances whose molecular weights and valencies are not precisely known cannot be included in this scheme (e.g., proteins). It will take some time for people to become accustomed to new ranges of values and nomenclatures (e.g., bilirubin 5·2 mg./100 ml. becomes 88·9 mol./litre; cholesterol 250 mg./100 ml. becomes 6·46 mmol./litre; and urea 73 mg./100 ml. becomes 12·2 mmol./litre). It is, therefore, even more important than ever that results from individual laboratories be read and used in the light of their particular methods of estimation and their accepted normal ranges for these methods.

With increasing automation, 12 simultaneous different estimations can be carried out on one blood sample, and this has encouraged screening programmes of the normal population. It is worth noting that if the normal range (95 per cent of results) is accepted, 1 in every 20 results may fall outside this range in normal subjects. This introduces yet another problem in the interpretation of results by clinicians.

Bristol,   R. D. E.
March, 1971

PREFACE TO THE FIRST EDITION

IN this book I have tried to provide an accurate summary of the ways in which various conditions affect many biochemical tests. The attempt has been made because I have found in clinical laboratory practice that junior medical staff tend to read too much or too little into the results returning to them from the laboratory. Inevitably, I have missed out many tests either because I consider them dangerous or useless, or because they have been superseded by better tests, which are included.

A static reading of a result reflects only poorly the dynamic changes occurring in the body. In particular, some of the tests which are included cannot be dealt with adequately in the form used in this book. This applies especially to routine electrolyte examinations. For example, the plasma sodium level can be within the normal range, but the total body sodium may be either depleted, normal, or in gross excess. The patient's clinical state must be considered with every result from the laboratory. Nothing could be more dangerous to the patient's welfare, or more damaging to clinical chemistry, than attempts at either 'blunderbuss' diagnosis using multitudes of tests, or attempts to 'make a firm diagnosis' from a single result.

I have also included tests which are not normally performed by many routine laboratories, either because they demonstrate interesting applied physiology, or because of the exciting possibilities of future advances implicit in these tests.

In fact, if this book serves only to irritate more people into a state of greater interest in clinical chemistry, then it will have performed a useful function.

Finally, I would recommend the following subjects for discussion between the clinician and the clinical biochemist: (1) Clinical cases ; (2) The methods of estimation used ; (3) The ranges of normal values recognized by the particular laboratory.

I am grateful to *Dr. G. K. McGowan*, Consultant Chemical Pathologist, United Bristol Hospitals, for helpful advice and criticisms, and also for information on various subjects ; to *Dr. J. M. Naish*, Consultant Physician, Bristol Clinical Area, for advice and encouragement ; and to *Mr. W. B. Yeoman*, Biochemist, Frenchay Hospital, for helpful advice, criticisms, and information on various subjects.

Bristol,   R. D. E.
December, 1959

DEFINITION

The Equivalent Weight of a substance is that weight of it which will combine with or displace 1 g. atom of hydrogen or 8 g. atoms of oxygen. A milliequivalent of the substance is therefore 1/1000 of this weight, e.g. :—

	Equivalent weight	1 mEq.
Sodium	23 g.	23 mg.
Potassium	39 g.	39 mg.
Chloride	35·5 g.	35·5 mg.
Bicarbonate	2·24 l.	2·24 ml. CO_2 at N.T.P.
Calcium	20 g.	20 mg.

BIOCHEMICAL VALUES IN CLINICAL MEDICINE

The Results following Pathological or Physiological Change

BY

ROBERT DUNCAN EASTHAM

B.A. (Cantab.), M.D. (Cantab.), F.R.C.Path., D.C.P., Dipl. Path.

Consultant Pathologist to the Frenchay Group of Hospitals, Bristol; Lately Consultant Pathologist to the Newcastle General Hospital, Newcastle upon Tyne

FOURTH EDITION

BRISTOL: JOHN WRIGHT & SONS LTD.

1971

BY THE SAME AUTHOR

Clinical Hæmatology
A Laboratory Guide to Clinical Diagnosis
Clinical Pathology in Mental Retardation
(R. D. Eastham and J. Jancar)

First edition, January, 1960
Reprinted, August, 1961
Second edition, July, 1963
Reprinted, June, 1965
Third edition, May, 1967
Reprinted, December, 1968
Fourth edition, June, 1971

Italian edition, November, 1961
Greek edition, 1964
Spanish edition, 1968
German edition, May, 1970

Distribution by Sole Agents:
United States of America: The Williams & Wilkins Company, Baltimore
Canada: The Macmillan Company of Canada Ltd., Toronto

ISBN 0 7236 0298 0

PRINTED IN GREAT BRITAIN BY JOHN WRIGHT & SONS LTD.,
AT THE STONEBRIDGE PRESS, BRISTOL BS4 5NU

BIOCHEMICAL VALUES IN CLINICAL MEDICINE

ACIDITY OF URINE

ACIDIFICATION TEST.—After oral ammonium chloride, 0·1 g. per kg. body-weight, in water, urine specimens are collected and stored under liquid paraffin until they can be examined in the laboratory. Delay should be minimal.

Normally the urine pH falls below 5·3 within 3 hours, and the urine ammonium excretion increases. The rate of urine ammonium excretion is inversely proportional to the urine pH. Normally under these conditions more than 1·5 mEq. of ammonium is excreted per hour; less than 0·5 mEq. per hour suggests renal tubular damage.

In generalized renal disease the urine pH falls normally, but ammonium excretion is scanty. In renal tubular acidosis the urine pH does not decrease, and the rate of ammonium excretion is low, but normal in relation to the urine pH. Defect in urinary acidification has been described in sickle-cell anæmia.

After 6 g. of oral ammonium chloride, a normal adult would excrete 70–160 mEq. of ammonium in the urine per 24 hr.

N.B.—**It is very dangerous to give ammonium chloride to patients suffering from liver failure or hepatic cirrhosis.**

REFERENCES.—Davies, H. E. F., and Wrong, O. (1957), *Lancet*, **2**, 625; Kong, H. H. P., and Alleyne, G. A. O. (1968), *Ibid.*, **2**, 954.

TITRATABLE ACIDITY.—The titratable acidity represents the sum of the organic acids and sodium dihydrogen phosphate excreted in the urine. Added to the ammonium excreted in the urine, it gives a measure of the extent to which the body is able to conserve sodium and potassium while excreting excess anions and hydrogen ions.

N.B.—**This is not a useful clinical test.**

TOTAL FIXED BASE OF URINE

This consists of the total urine excretion of sodium, potassium, magnesium, and calcium per day. It is not a useful estimation.

ADRENAL INHIBITION TESTS

In a normal person cortisone inhibits adrenal cortical activity, probably by inhibiting the formation of ACTH.

Pathological.—

1. *Virilizing States.*—Daily administration of 200 mg. cortisone acetate (orally or i.m.) for 2–5 days to those cases with abnormally raised 17-oxosteroid excretion gives the following results:—

   a. Adrenal hyperplasia. The daily urine output of 17-oxosteroids is reduced.

    b. Adrenal adenoma ⎫   The daily urine output of
    c. Adrenal carcinoma ⎬   17-oxosteroids is unaffected.

2. *Cushing's Syndrome.*—Following daily administration orally of 10 mg. of 9-alpha-fluorohydrocortisone, the daily urine output of 17-oxogenic steroids is greatly reduced.

Recently it has been found that 9-alpha-fluoro-16-alpha-methyl-prednisolone (dexamethasone) can be used. 0·5 mg. 6-hourly for 8 doses suppresses normal adrenals, but not hyperplastic adrenals (whatever cause). 2·0 mg. 6-hourly for 8 doses suppresses benign adrenal hyperplasia but not malignant hyperactivity.

REFERENCE.—Sprague, R. G., Weeks, R. E., Priestley, J. T., and Salassa, R. M. (1961), *Modern Trends in Endocrinology* (Ed. Gardiner-Hill), p. 87. London: Butterworth.

ALCOHOL IN BLOOD AND URINE

Subclinical intoxication, 0–100 mg./100 ml.
Critical level of obvious intoxication, probably 150 mg./100 ml.
Gross intoxication, 200 mg./100 ml.
Stupor, more than 300 mg./100 ml.

$$\left(\frac{\text{mg./litre}}{46} = \text{mmol./litre.}\right)$$

Urine concentration is usually about one-third higher than the blood concentration. Peak urine output of alcohol is reached 2 hours after ingestion. Recently estimation of the breath alcohol has been used as a measure of the blood alcohol concentration.

There is direct correlation between alveolar air alcohol concentration and arterial blood alcohol concentration.

REFERENCES.—Walls, H. J. (1958), *Brit. med. J.*, 1, 1442; Editorial (1966), *Ibid.*, 1, 184.

N.B.—**There are usually legal implications involved.**

ALDOLASE IN SERUM

The enzyme catalyses the reaction:—
    1 molecule of fructose diphosphate → 2 molecules of triose phosphate.
The highest tissue concentrations of the enzyme are found in heart muscle and skeletal muscle.

Normal Range.—2–9·6 units/ml. serum (1·5–7·2 μmol./min./litre). Red blood-cells contain aldolase in concentrations 150 times higher than the normal serum level.

Physiological.—
Increase.—Normal newborn serum and red-cell levels are higher than the equivalent maternal levels for the first 48 hours after birth. Normal adult levels are reached by puberty.

Pathological.—
Increase.—
    1. *Myocardial Infarction.*—Serum level rises after 3 hours to a peak by 24 hours (2–15 ×normal), falling to

normal by 4–7 days. There is a semiquantitative relationship between the amount of myocardial necrosis and the peak level in the serum.

2. *Skeletal Muscle Damage.*—

   a. Progressive muscle dystrophy. (Affected muscles showing true hypertrophy, pseudohypertrophy, or atrophy.) Serum level increases in the early stages to 10–15 × normal in 90 per cent of cases. In pseudohypertrophic muscular dystrophy the serum levels are increased before there are obvious clinical signs of the disease. Levels in serum are higher in affected children than in adults in whom muscular dystrophy is developing for the first time. In the later and terminal stages serum aldolase levels are normal. Dystrophic muscle has an abnormally low aldolase content.

   b. Gangrene affecting muscle.

   c. Erb-Duchenne brachial plexus paralysis, i.e., C.5 nerve torn at birth. Serum level rises in the early stages, falling to normal later. This occurs in any primary neurogenic muscular atrophy.

   d. Dermatomyositis. Normal or moderately increased serum levels are found. Where the serum level is increased, treatment with steroids will reduce the level to normal.

   e. Paroxysmal myoglobinuria. Raised serum levels related to muscle destruction.

   Whenever there is rapid destruction of skeletal muscle there is an increase in serum aldolase accompanied by parallel rises in serum lactic dehydrogenase, transaminases, and phosphohexoseisomerase, since these enzymes are also released from muscle cells.

   Any destruction or wasting of muscle results in increased urine creatine output. In poliomyelitis, myotonic dystrophy, and other muscle disorders of nervous origin the serum aldolase is normal. In muscle wasting following severance of a nerve the serum aldolase shows a transient rise.

   f. Carbenoxolone therapy.

3. *Liver Damage.*—

   a. Acute hepatitis.

   b. Acute alcoholic psychosis (? due to associated liver damage).

   c. Poisoning with carbon tetrachloride and other liver poisons.

   d. Secondary carcinoma invading the liver.

   e. Glycogen storage disease.

4. *Acute Pancreatitis.*

5. *Megaloblastic Anæmia* (serum levels up to 17 × normal may occur).

6. *Hæmolytic Anæmia.*—Serum levels increased if severe.

7. *Pulmonary Embolism.*—Moderate increase with no sharp peak, cf. myocardial infarction.

8. *Carcinomatosis.*—Variable rises in serum levels may be found. Successful remission in carcinoma of prostate produced by œstrogens is reflected by a fall in the

serum level towards normal. In carcinomatosis the serum levels of aldolase and phosphohexoseisomerase are roughly parallel.

9. Cortisone and ACTH both cause the serum aldolase level to rise in experimental animals. ? similar effect in man.

10. *Tetanus.* Very high serum levels found in severe cases.

   N.B.—The serum aldolase changes in so many different conditions that it is really only useful either in the detection of cases of muscular dystrophy in the early stages of the disease or to measure response to treatment in carcinomatosis. (Probably serum phosphohexoseisomerase is a better parameter in these latter cases.)

REFERENCES.—Sibley, J. A., and Lehninger, A. L. (1949), *J. biol. Chem.*, **177**, 859; Volk, B. W., Losner, S., Aronson, S. M., and Lew, H. (1956), *Amer. J. med. Sci.*, **232**, 38; Thompson, R. A., and Vignos, P. J. (1959), *Arch. intern. Med.*, **103**, 551; Patel, A. A., and Rao, S. S. (1966), *Amer. J. med. Sci.*, **251**, 290.

ALDOLASE IN CEREBROSPINAL FLUID

Pathological.—

Increase.—

1. Niemann-Pick disease.
2. Infantile amaurotic familial idiocy.

ALDOSTERONE IN URINE

The hormone aldosterone is formed in the glomerulosa cells of the adrenal cortex. Normal excretion in the urine—up to 15 μg./24 hr. as aldosterone and its 18-glucuronide (equivalent to about 10 per cent of the adrenal secretion rate).

Physiological.—

Increase.—

1. Low sodium in the diet, with adequate potassium, especially if ACTH is given also.
2. Excessive sodium loss, with adequate potassium intake, e.g., after sweating.
3. After administration of potassium salts.
4. Normal pregnancy in third trimester.

Decrease.—

1. Excessive water intake.
2. Excess hypertonic saline infusion.
3. Low potassium intake.

Pathological.—

Increase.—

1. Primary hyperaldosteronism.—
   a. Adrenal adenoma.
   b. Adrenal carcinoma.

N.B.—**In the presence of a low plasma potassium concentration, aldosterone excretion may be normal.**

2. Secondary hyperaldosteronism.—
   a. Excessive sodium loss.—
      i. Severe sweating.
      ii. Sodium diuresis.
      iii. Post-hæmorrhage.
      iv. Post-operation.

v. Salt-losing nephritis.
  b. Œdematous states.—
    i. Cardiac failure.
    ii. Hepatic cirrhosis.
    iii. Nephrosis.
  c. Bartter's syndrome.

Decrease.—
1. Addison's disease. The adrenal cortex is progressively destroyed.
2. Excessive infusion of either hypertonic saline, glucose solution, or rectal water (i.e., expansion of the plasma-volume).
3. Smaller increase than normal in eclampsia.
4. Congenital adrenal hyperplasia.

N.B.—The production of aldosterone, in cases other than adrenal tumour cases, appears to be related to the effective plasma-volume. It is not apparently directly controlled by the pituitary gland.

REFERENCE.—Thorn, G. W., Ross, E. J., Crabbe, J., and Van'T Hoff W. (1957), *Brit. med. J.*, **2**, 955.

ALKAPTONURIA

This is a rare condition inherited via a recessive Mendelian character. Excessive amounts of homogentisic acid are excreted in the urine. The urine darkens on standing, especially if it is alkaline. Homogentisic acid is an intermediate substance formed during conversion of phenylalanine to tyrosine; its output in the urine is proportional to the amount of protein in the diet.

Theories.—
1. Homogentisic acid is manufactured by the renal tubular cells.
2. Renal tubular cells extract traces of homogentisic acid present in the blood in these cases, and actively secrete it.

Both these theories are compatible with the finding that the renal threshold for this substance is extremely low.

AMINO-ACIDS

AMINO-ACIDS IN BLOOD.—
Normal Range.—In plasma, 4·3–7·7 mg./100 ml. (as nitrogen). Higher readings are obtained with serum since amino-acids are liberated during clotting. The red blood-cells normally contain twice as much as the plasma.

Physiological.—
  Increase.—After a protein-containing meal the plasma level rises. The plasma level returns to the pre-prandial concentration within 4 hours.
  Decrease.—The plasma level falls after glucose ingestion or insulin administration.
    The plasma level also falls after growth-hormone or androgen ingestion. Presumably protein synthesis is stimulated.

N.B.—In starvation the blood level does not usually fall below the normal fasting level (i.e., the level is maintained at the expense of body protein).

Pathological.—

Increase.—

1. Liver disease.—
   a. Acute yellow atrophy. The amino-acid level in the plasma is roughly proportional to the degree of liver damage. The greatest increase is in methionine and tyrosine.
   b. Fatal liver poisoning with phosphorus, phenylhydrazine, carbon tetrachloride, or chloroform.
   c. Kwashiorkor. There is an increase in beta-aminoisobutyric acid. During recovery with liver regeneration, the predominant amino-acid is ethanolamine.
   d. Severe yellow fever.
   e. Eclampsia.
   f. Cœliac disease and idiopathic steatorrhœa (if liver damage is also present).
2. Severe burns. Peptides derived from the burnt tissues appear in the plasma.
3. Severe shock.
4. After hæmorrhage (especially gastro-intestinal bleeding).
5. Diabetes mellitus in ketosis (probably associated with gluconeogenesis).
6. Slight increases have been reported in acute infections, hyperthyroidism, congestive cardiac failure, some cases of anæmia, and after the administration of corticotrophin or cortisone.

Decrease.—

1. Nephrosis.
2. Kwashiorkor. Reduced to 45 per cent of normal.

The isolated estimation of the amino-acid content of the blood is not often useful. Severe liver damage is more easily detectable by other means, but an abnormally raised plasma level could possibly assist in the detection of acute yellow atrophy of the liver.

The protein ingestion test of West has been used in the diagnosis of fibrous cystic disease of the pancreas in children. Its extension for the detection of chronic pancreatitis in adults has been found unsatisfactory by the author.

Probably chromatographic separation and identification of amino-acids showing abnormal increase in the plasma is useful occasionally, e.g., in liver disease. Generally the more important changes in the plasma amino-acids are reflected in the urinary chromatogram.

REFERENCES.—Folin, O. (1922), *J. biol. Chem.*, 51, 377 ; Smith, I. (1958), *Chromatographic Techniques*. London : Heinemann.

AMINO-ACIDS IN URINE.—

The daily urine amino-acid output in normal adults is about 1·1 g. as free amino-acids and about 2 g. as conjugated amino-acids, with wide variation between individuals. This variation may be caused by diet, genetic differences, pregnancy, etc.

Physiological.—
1. On a high meat diet, excess histidine and methyl histidine are excreted.
2. In starvation excess beta-amino-isobutyric acid is excreted.
3. During normal pregnancy increased amounts of histidine and threonine are excreted, returning to normal during lactation.
4. In full-term and premature babies increased amounts of glycine, alanine, threonine, serine, asparagine, glutamine, cystine, glutamic acid, and proline are excreted in excess in the urine.

N.B.—**Patients treated with a mixture of D- and L-amino-acids show a gross amino-aciduria, since the dextrorotatory forms of the amino-acids are only poorly utilized by the body and are rapidly lost in the urine. Patients having intravenous infusions of protein hydrolysates may show amino-aciduria, presumably due to incomplete utilization.**

Pathological.—
1. *Pure 'Overflow' Amino-aciduria.—*
   Liver Disease.—
   i. Massive liver necrosis.
   ii. Advanced cirrhosis of the liver.
      In both these conditions the amount of amino-acids present in the plasma, cerebrospinal fluid, and urine is proportional to the degree of liver damage.
      The appearance and amounts of cystine, beta-amino-isobutyric acid, and ethanolamine are a useful indication of liver damage. Glutamine may appear in the urine if the patient has been treated with glutamic acid.
   iii. Post-anæsthetic transitory cystinuria.
   iv. Liver regeneration. Predominantly an increase in ethanolamine.
   v. Kwashiorkor. Increased beta-amino-isobutyric acid and ethanolamine.
2. *Unclassified.—*
   *a. Untreated Pernicious Anæmia.—*There is amino-aciduria with an excess excretion of taurine, especially if there is associated subacute combined degeneration of the spinal cord. Amino-aciduria does not occur in other megalo-blastic anæmias.
   *b. March Hæmoglobinuria.—*Cystine and beta-amino-isobutyric acid may appear.
   *c. Acute Intermittent Porphyria.—*Urine contains delta-amino-lævulinic acid.
   *d. Alactasia.—*Urine contains lactose plus amino-acids after a lactose-containing diet.
   *e. Cachexia.—*The predominant amino-acid appearing in the urine is beta-amino-isobutyric acid.
   f. Glycogen Storage Disease.
   *g. Severe Diabetic Ketosis.—*The predominant amino-acids in the urine are leucine and lysine.

REFERENCES.—Harris, H., and Milne, M. D. (1964), *Biochemical Disorders*, 2nd ed. (Ed. Thompson, R. H. S., and King, E. J.), Ch. 18, p. 743. London: Churchill; Milne, M. D. (1964), *Brit. med. J.*, 1, 327 (156 references); Eastham, R. D., and Jancar, J. (1968), *Clinical Pathology in Mental Retardation.* Bristol: Wright.

HEREDITARY CONDITIONS WITH ASSOCIATED AMINO-ACIDURIA

Clinical Condition	Amino-acidæmia	Amino-aciduria
Carbamyl phosphate synthetase deficiency	Glycine	Glycine
Ornithine transcarbamylase deficiency	No increase	Moderate amino-aciduria with increased glutamin
Citrullinuria	Citrulline	Citrulline
Argininosuccinic aciduria	Argininosuccinic acid + citrulline	Argininosuccinic acid
Arginase deficiency	Arginine	Gross amino-aciduria with excess arginine
Congenital lysine intolerance	Lysine with moderate increase in arginine, glutamine, ornithine	Lysine, with ornithine ethanolamine, gamma-aminobutyric acid
Phenylketonuria	Phenylalanine	Phenylalanine + keto-derivatives
Tyrosinæmia	Tyrosine, with increased methionine in acute attacks	p-Hydroxyphenyl derivatives
Hartnup disease	Abnormally low plasma tryptophan	Generalized amino-aciduria with specific pattern
Tryptophanuria	Tryptophan	Tryptophan
Indolylacroyl glycinuria	No increase described	Indolylacroyl glycine
Maple-syrup urine disease	Valine, leucine, isoleucine	Valine, leucine, isoleucin
Hypervalinæmia	Valine	Valine
Isovaleric acidæmia	Isovaleric acid (essential amino-acids depressed)	Isovaleric acid
Hypermethioninæmia	Methionine + tyrosine	Amino-aciduria with specific pattern
Oast-house syndrome	No increase	Phenylalanine, tyrosine methionine plus variou keto-acids
Homocystinuria	Methionine + homocystine	Homocystine plus othe sulphur-containing substances
Cystathioninuria	Methionine after methionine load	Cystathionine
Cystinosis	Free cystine in leucocytes increased	Amino-aciduria with increased cystine
Cystinuria	Normal	Cystine, lysine, arginin ornithine
Sulphite oxidase deficiency	No report	Cysteine derivative
Histidinæmia	Histidine	Histidine plus imidazol derivatives
Hereditary orotic aciduria		Orotic acid
Hyperglycinæmia with hyperglycinuria (ketotic variety)	Glycine, with moderate increases in branched amino-acids + methionine	Glycine
Hyperglycinæmia with hyperglycinuria (non-ketotic)	Glycine	Glycine
Monilethrix	Glutamic acid	Variable
Hypersarcosinæmia	Sarcosine	Sarcosine
Oculo-otocerebrorenal syndrome	Alpha-aminobutyric acid	Alpha-aminobutyric acid
Hyperbeta-alaninæmia	Alanine + gamma-iso-butyric acid	Beta-alanine, beta-amin isobutyric acid, gamm aminobutyric acid
Familial hyperprolinæmia, Type I	Proline	Proline, glycine, hydrox proline
Familial hyperprolinæmia, Type II	Proline	Proline + delta-pyrroline 5-carboxylic acid
Hydroxyprolinæmia	Hydroxyproline	Hydroxyproline (free)
Oculocerebrorenal syndrome	Normal	Multiple amino-aciduria
Methylmalonic aciduria	Normal	Methylmalonic acid
A-beta-lipoproteinæmia	Normal	Non-specific

Clinical Condition	Amino-acidæmia	Amino-aciduria
Amaurotic familial idiocy	Normal	Carnosine and derivatives of histidine may be found
Hereditary fructose intolerance	General increase	General amino-aciduria
Galactosæmia		Amino-aciduria
Familial lactic acidosis		Moderate amino-aciduria
Hepatolenticular degeneration	Normal	Generalized amino-aciduria

ALANINE AMINOTRANSFERASE AND ASPARTATE AMINOTRANSFERASE

TRANSAMINASE IN SERUM.—Two serum transaminases are estimated in clinical practice, namely serum glutamic-oxalacetic transaminase (SGOT) and serum glutamic-pyruvate transaminase (SGPT).

Normal Range.—

1. Serum GOT—Less than 40 units per ml. (2–20 i.u./litre).
2. Serum GPT—Less than 30 units per ml. (2–15 i.u./litre).

REFERENCES.—(SGOT) Karmen, A., Wroblewski, F., and La Due, J. S. (1955), *J. clin. Invest.*, 34, 126; (SGPT) Wroblewski, F., and La Due, J. S. (1956), *Proc. Soc. exper. Biol., N.Y.*, 91, 569.

GLUTAMIC-OXALACETIC TRANSAMINASE IN SERUM (ASPARTATE AMINOTRANSFERASE).—

Physiological.—

Increase.—The SGOT is raised in the normal newborn. Normal adult levels are reached by 7 years.

Pathological.—

Increase.—Normally almost all the enzyme is intracellular. Following any injury to, or death, of physiologically active cells, the enzyme is released into the circulation, i.e., it can be used as a measure of cell damage rather than cell function. Equilibration between plasma and interstitial fluid then follows within 6–18 hours, i.e., the serum rise is not as great as would be expected from total enzyme released from damaged tissue.

1. *Heart.*—
    a. Myocardial infarction: The SGOT level increases about 4 hours after an infarction, and persists at an abnormally raised level for about 3 days. SGOT also rises in acute congestive failure related to centrilobular liver necrosis and congestion. A normal SGOT excludes cardiac infarction *if* the time of sampling is correct.
    b. Acute rheumatic carditis: Serum level related to severity in the early stages.
    c. Cardiac surgery: On the second day after operation the serum level is increased, falling to normal by the tenth day—e.g., after operation for pulmonary stenosis the SGOT is 7–8 × normal.
    d. After angiocardiography and passage of cardiac catheter.
    e. After external cardiac massage.
2. *Liver.*—
    a. Infective hepatitis: The serum level rises in the prodromal phases of the disease, increasing to a peak when the patient shows the greatest malaise and liver

tenderness. The rise in the enzyme is parallel with the rise in serum iron (cf. extrahepatic biliary obstruction). SGOT correlates well with the course of chronic hepatitis. The level is raised in non-icteric attacks.

b. Hepatic damage: Carbon tetrachloride and other liver poisons cause the SGOT to rise.

c. Infiltration of liver:—
   i. Carcinoma ⎫
   ii. Leukæmia ⎬ Cases may show an increase.
   iii. Lymphoma ⎭

d. Cholangitis.

e. Infectious mononucleosis: Maximal results by the second week, falling to normal by the fifth week.

f. Alcoholic debauch: SGOT rises afterwards.

g. Pulmonary infarction: SGOT rises later and slower than after cardiac infarction. Possibly related to associated congestive failure.

3. *Pancreas.*—Acute pancreatitis. No apparent correlation with: (a) Damage to pancreas, (b) Serum lipase, (c) Serum amylase, (d) Serum calcium, but there is direct correlation with the serum bilirubin level suggesting increase due to biliary obstruction.

4. *Trauma.*—
   a. Intestinal infarction.
   b. Intestinal surgery.
   c. Crush injury.
   d. Local irradiation injury.
   e. Carbon monoxide poisoning, from skeletal muscle, heart muscle, and brain.
   f. Following direct current countershock to convert arrhythmia to normal rhythm (from intercostal muscle damage).
   g. Severe heat stroke.
   h. Following intramuscular injection of ampicillin or carbenicillin, due to skeletal muscle damage.

5. *Other.*—
   a. Pseudohypertrophic muscular dystrophy: The enzyme is released from breaking down muscle. The SGOT levels tend to be increased in affected young children, and fall to normal in the later stages.
   b. Dermatomyositis: SGOT may be increased in the absence of clinical evidence of muscle wasting. Steroid therapy causes the level to fall towards normal. (In rheumatoid arthritis, discoid lupus erythematosus, scleroderma, and acrosclerosis, SGOT is normal.)
   c. Myoglobinuria.
   d. Gout: Increased levels have been reported in acute stages.
   e. Salicylate therapy, in heavy dosage: This may possibly be evidence of some liver damage.
   f. Status asthmaticus (? due to anoxic tissue damage).
   g. At onset of clofibrate therapy.

N.B.—The SGOT level is normal in chlorpromazine jaundice. Serum and plasma contain almost equal GOT activity, but platelets contain more GOT activity.

Blood hæmolysates contain ten times as much GOT as serum does. Therefore, unhæmolysed blood-samples are essential for analysis.

SGOT isoenzymes are not useful.

GLUTAMIC-PYRUVATE TRANSAMINASE IN SERUM (ALANINE AMINOTRANSFERASE).—

Physiological.—The SGPT is low in normal cord blood: the concentration gradually rises to a peak by the fifth day after birth in the infant.

REFERENCE.—Haug, H., and Kluge, A. (1965), *Klin. Wschr.*, **12**, 680.

Pathological.—
Increase.—
1. *Acute Hepatitis.*—A marked increase occurs, which is relatively greater than the rise in SGOT. Serum GPT superior to SGOT in detection of infective hepatitis. The level is raised in non-icteric attacks.
2. *Relapsing Cirrhosis of the Liver.*—There is a marked increase, associated with the rise in SGOT.
3. *Myocardial Infarction.*—Only a small increase occurs (cf. SGOT).
4. *Infectious Mononucleosis.*—Maximal by second week and normal by fifth week.
5. At onset of clofibrate therapy.

GLUTAMIC-OXALACETIC TRANSAMINASE IN CEREBRO-SPINAL FLUID.—

Increase.—
1. GOT increased for some days after cerebral infarction or cerebrovascular accident without a corresponding rise in CSF GPT.
2. Slight increase with prolapsed intervertebral disk.
3. After cerebral anoxia in hypoxia, GOT leaks from cerebral tissues into CSF.
4. Carcinoma metastases in central nervous system. (Normal results with primary CNS tumours.)

REFERENCE.—Davies-Jones, G. A. B. (1969), *J. Neurol. Neurosurg. Psychiat.*, **32**, 324.

AMMONIA

AMMONIA IN BLOOD.—

Normal Range.—

Normal arterial plasma $= <10\,\mu g./100$ ml.

Normal venous plasma $= <30\,\mu g./100$ ml.

Normal blood draining gastro-intestinal tract $=150\,\mu g./100$ ml.

$$\left(\frac{\mu g./\text{litre}}{17} = \mu\text{mol./litre.}\right)$$

Normally only traces of ammonia are present in the blood. The liver removes it as rapidly as it is formed. Ammonia increases rapidly in blood samples on standing. It also increases in venous blood after muscular exercise. In health and disease the distribution of ammonia between red cells and plasma is nearly equal to the distribution of hydrogen ions between red cells and plasma. The patient's mental state is impaired when the arterial plasma concentration exceeds 100 μg./100 ml.

Pathological.—

Increase.—

1. Hepatectomy in the experimental animal.
2. Acute hepatic necrosis.
3. Terminal portal cirrhosis.
   a. Agonal.
   b. After high protein diet.
   c. After oral resins in the ammonium phase, used to control œdema and ascites.
   d. After ammonium chloride ingestion.
   e. After portacaval shunt.
4. Congenital enzyme deficiencies.
   a. Carbamyl phosphate synthetase.
   b. Ornithine transcarbamylase.
   c. Argininosuccinate synthetase.
   d. Congenital lysine intolerance.
5. Hæmorrhagic shock.
6. Erythroblastosis fœtalis.
7. Emphysema.

When confusion or coma with a raised blood ammonia level is provoked either by a high protein diet or ammonium chloride, the prognosis is grave. It is possible that uptake of ammonia by the brain causes alpha-ketoglutarate to be converted to glutamate; hence any deficiency in the rate of formation of alpha-ketoglutarate would interrupt the Krebs citric acid cycle.

Note.—The liver is the site of:—

1. Deamination of amino-acids.
2. Deamination of adenylic acid.
3. Synthesis of glutamine.

The blood ammonia level may not be increased in all cases of hepatic coma. The estimation of blood ammonia is not usually performed by routine laboratories. Some samples of heparin used as anticoagulant contain significant amounts of ammonia.

REFERENCE.—Fenton, J. C. B., and Williams, A. H. (1968), *J. clin. Path.*, **21**, 14.

AMMONIA IN URINE.—

Normal Average Excretion.—20–70 mEq./24 hr., i.e., equivalent to the excretion of 200–700 ml. of N/10 acid neutralized by ammonia. The maximum rate of ammonium excretion is about 400 mEq. per day.

Ammonia is produced in the distal renal tubules, by the action of glutaminase on glutamine (60 per cent) and by the

Glutamine → glutamic
$$\text{acid} + NH_3 \searrow$$
$$NH_4 + NaCl \rightleftharpoons NH_4Cl + NaHCO_3$$
$$H_2CO_3 \rightarrow HCO_3 + H^+ \nearrow$$

deamination of other amino-acids (40 per cent). The liberated ammonia immediately combines with hydrogen ions derived from ionizing carbonic acid, to form ammonium ions. These latter are exchanged for sodium and potassium ions in the urine in the tubules.

This production of ammonia ions allows the excretion of excess anions and hydrogen ions without the corresponding loss of fixed base (sodium and potassium). The logarithm of the rate of ammonia excretion is inversely proportional to the pH of the urine. The peak of ammonia excretion is only reached about four days after the onset of acidosis, and it subsides equally slowly after the stimulus ceases.

Physiological.—

Increase (Acid Urines).—

1. High meat diet (i.e., daily anion excess).
2. Raised mineral acid intake, e.g., in the form of salts such as ammonium chloride.
3. Low carbohydrate diet.
4. Starvation, i.e., body protein breakdown.
5. Normal pregnancy. Moderate acidosis develops normally in the final three months.

Decrease (Alkaline Urines).—

1. Vegetarian diet.
2. Increased alkali intake, e.g., sodium bicarbonate.

Pathological.—

Increase.—

1. Metabolic acidosis.
   a. In diabetes mellitus during prolonged ketosis, the maximum rate of excretion is attained.
   b. Starvation.
   c. Dehydration.
   d. Prolonged vomiting (with associated achlorhydria and ketosis).
   e. Prolonged diarrhœa.
2. Respiratory acidosis.
3. Potassium depletion (possibly due to associated intracellular acidosis).
4. Sodium depletion (possibly due to retention of sodium and chloride ions by the renal tubules).
5. Fanconi syndrome.
6. Primary hyperaldosteronism (possibly due to hormone action on the renal tubule cells or possibly due to the associated potassium depletion).

Decrease.—

1. Metabolic alkalosis, e.g., excessive alkali intake.
2. Respiratory alkalosis.
3. Nephritis with damage to the distal renal tubules.
4. Addison's disease.

N.B.—**Urea-splitting organisms in the bladder or in the urine after collection will produce falsely high levels of urine ammonia.**

In practice, the estimation of urine ammonia is mainly useful after oral ammonium chloride, in parallel with urine pH measurements. This gives a measure of ammonia production by the distal renal tubules in response to induced acidosis. (Urine acidification test.)

REFERENCE.—King, E. J. (1956), *Micro-analysis in Medical Biochemistry*, 3rd ed. London : Churchill.

AMYLASE

AMYLASE IN SERUM.—

Normal Range.—80–180 Somogyi units/100 ml.; 3–10 Wohlgemuth units/1 ml.; 86–268 i.u./litre.

Physiological.—

The blood level in any normal individual appears to be fairly constant. The concentration in infants' blood is very low for the first two months; then it increases to reach normal adult levels by the end of the first year of life. Serum amylase levels fall after glucose, fructose, glucagon, or insulin.

The site of formation of all the blood amylase is not known. Removal of pancreas and salivary glands in dogs produces no marked change in the blood level.

Pathological.—

Increase.—

1. *Pancreatic Disorders:—*

    a. Acute pancreatitis. The highest levels are found during the period 5–12 hours after the onset of the attack, after which the blood level may rapidly fall to normal (cf. blood lipase).

    Serum levels of > 1000 Somogyi units/100 ml. very strongly suggest a diagnosis of acute pancreatitis.

    b. Acute exacerbation of chronic pancreatitis. Again, the elevated blood level is only transitory.

    c. Perforated peptic ulcer, particularly if the pancreas is involved.

    d. Postgastrectomy   } Levels over 1000 units/
    e. Afferent loop obstruction } 100 ml. may be found.

    f. Cholecystitis.

    g. Calculous obstruction of the pancreatic duct.

    h. Opiates, codeine, and methyl choline (by causing spasm of the sphincter of the pancreatic duct).

    i. Secretin, pancreozymin, and methyl choline all stimulate gland secretion. In the presence of a partial or complete block of the pancreatic duct, the blood level tends to rise.

    j. Corticosteroid therapy may occasionally precipitate acute pancreatitis.

    k. Abnormal amylase, a macromolecule of molecular weight 200,000 with no loss in urine.

    l. Following scorpion sting.

2. *Salivary Gland Disease.—*

    a. Mumps. Apart from involvement of the salivary glands, the pancreas may also be affected.

    b. Suppurative parotitis.

    c. Calculous obstruction of the salivary duct.

3. *Other Conditions.—*

    a. Methanol poisoning.

    b. After gross ethanol intake (in the chronic alcoholic). The mechanism whereby the blood amylase increases in these two conditions (*a* and *b*) is not known.

    c. Renal disease. It is possible that renal disease associated with poor excretion of the enzyme in the urine may cause a slight elevation in the blood level. In the presence of oliguria, the serum amylase may rise to "diagnostic" levels.

    d. About 10 per cent of cases of severe accidental hypothermia develop acute pancreatitis.

    e. Chronic malabsorption with intestinal villous atrophy. ˣ

    f. Pancreatitis developing in children on steroid therapy.

N.B.—Only the finding of a gross increase in the blood level (at least 500 Somogyi units/100 ml. or 100 Wohlgemuth units/ 1 ml.) is significant when a diagnosis of acute pancreatitis is considered.

Decrease.—

1. Gross rapid destruction of the pancreas in necrotic pancreatitis. This is an unusual mode of presentation of "acute pancreatitis".
2. Hepatitis.
3. Cholecystitis (some cases).
4. Severe burns.
5. Severe thyrotoxicosis.
6. Toxæmia of pregnancy.
7. Poisoning with carbon tetrachloride, barbiturates, or arsenic.
8. Possibly in some cases of congestive cardiac failure.
9. Possibly in some cases of diabetes mellitus.
10. Adrenocortical stress.
11. Propylthiouracil therapy.
12. Convalescent period after acute pancreatitis.

It is possible that liver damage associated with the above conditions may cause a fall in the blood amylase. Obviously destruction of the pancreas might be expected to produce a lower level in the blood. In general, the finding of an abnormally low blood level is of no clinical significance, except possibly where clinical signs indicate a severe abdominal catastrophe compatible with necrotic pancreatitis.

REFERENCES.—Machella, T. E. (1955), *Arch. intern. Med.*, **96**, 322 (Review of methods); McGowan, G. K., and Wills, M. R. (1964), *Brit. med. J.*, **1**, 160; Berk, J. E., Kizu, H., Wilding, P., and Seary, R. L. (1967), *New Engl. J. Med.*, **277**, 941; Ceska, M., Brown, B., and Birath, K. (1969), *Clin. chim. Acta*, **26**, 445; Bartholomew, C. (1970), *Brit. med. J.*, **1**, 666.

AMYLASE IN URINE.—

Normal Excretion Rate.—8000–30,000 Wohlgemuth units/ 24 hr.; average, 2–50 Wohlgemuth units/1 ml.; 127–1310 i.u./ litre.

Reduced Excretion.—

1. Liver diseases (some cases).
2. Renal disease (some cases).

Normal Excretion.—Normal values may be obtained during an attack of acute pancreatitis, following massive acute destruction of the pancreas.

Increased Excretion.—

1. Very high values are found during the first 24 hours of an attack of acute pancreatitis. In the absence of renal disease, the urine amylase is always raised in cases of acute pancreatitis when the plasma amylase level is increased. Although the blood level usually falls to normal within 3–4 days, the urine excretion may remain increased for 7–10 days or more.

2. Moderately high levels may be found in:—
   a. Duodenal ulcer perforating on to the pancreas.
   b. Stone in the common bile-duct.
   c. Carcinoma involving the common bile-duct.
   d. Stone in the pancreatic duct.
   e. Carcinoma of the pancreas.
3. Salivary gland disease.—
   a. Mumps.
   b. Suppurative parotitis.
   c. Stone in the salivary duct.

REFERENCE.—Saxon, E. I., Hinkley, W. C., Vogel, W. C., and Zieve, L. (1957), *Arch. intern. Med.*, **99**, 607.

ANGIOTENSIN II IN BLOOD

Normal Range.—
Arterial blood.—$2 \cdot 4 \pm 1 \cdot 2$ ng./100 ml.
Venous blood.—50–75 per cent of arterial blood concentration.
The estimation is available at a few centres, using a specific radioimmunoassay.
Pathological.—
Increase.—
   1. Essential hypertension.
   2. Other forms of hypertension.
Decrease.—
   1. Conn's syndrome (primary hyperaldosteronism).
   2. Anephric patients.

REFERENCE.—Catt, K. J., Cain, M. D., Zimmet, P. Z., and Cran, E. (1969), *Brit. med. J.*, **1**, 819.

ANTIDIURETIC HORMONE (ADH) IN PLASMA

Normal Range.—
Adult males.—$0 \cdot 04$–$0 \cdot 85$ microunit/ml.
Adult females.—$0 \cdot 15$–$0 \cdot 60$ microunit/ml.
Pregnant females.—$0 \cdot 12$–$0 \cdot 50$ microunit/ml.
Pathological.—
*Increase.—*Inappropriate secretion of antidiuretic hormone. "Normal" levels of ADH are found when there should be none, or increased plasma levels.
Decrease.—
   1. Congestive cardiac failure.
   2. Nephrotic syndrome.
The value of this estimation has not yet been established.

REFERENCE.—Gupta, K. K. (1968), *Brit. med. J.*, **4**, 185.

BASAL METABOLIC RATE

Normal Range.—
   1. Aub and Du Bois: − 20 per cent to + 5 per cent.
   2. Robertson and Reid: − 15 per cent to + 15 per cent. (This standard is preferred.)
Because of the bulky apparatus and the difficult techniques involved in direct calorimetry, the basal metabolic rate (BMR) is calculated from the results of indirect calorimetry. Calorie output under basal conditions is estimated from oxygen

uptake. It is assumed that for each litre of oxygen consumed, 4·8 calories are produced (respiratory quotient of 0·82). From measurements of body height and weight, the body surface area is calculated, and from the body surface area and the oxygen uptake the basal metabolic rate is calculated.

It is essential that:—

1. The patient should not be taking any thyroid stimulating or thyroid depressing drugs.
2. The test should be performed after a twelve-hour fast, and at rest in peaceful surroundings.
3. The patient be given a practice test on the previous day, to accustom him to the procedure.

Physiology.—

1. Children's BMRs are greater than those of adults by + 25 per cent. The surface area/body-weight ratio is greater in children. It is difficult to estimate the BMR in a child under 12 years of age.
2. Adult male BMRs average +7 per cent more than average adult female BMRs.
3. In normal pregnancy the BMR is increased in the last trimester, and also during lactation.
4. The BMR falls normally in old people by as much as 20 per cent.
5. Obesity. Increase in body-surface area without increase in oxygen consumption results in reduced BMR.

Technical Faults leading to Falsely Raised Results.—

1. Excessive anxiety. This may be alleviated to some extent by a trial test on the previous day.
2. Ill-fitting mouthpiece.
3. Absence of teeth (poor grip on the mouthpiece).
4. Perforated ear-drum, leading to air leak.
5. External temperature change, if marked.
6. Moderate exercise by the patient.
7. Ingestion of food by the patient prior to the test.
8. Emotional disturbance of the patient.
9. After smoking, in some cases.

Pathological.—

Increase.—

1. Hyperthyroidism—the rise in the BMR is proportional to toxicity. The BMR may increase to + 75 per cent or more. It falls after a 10-day course of potassium iodide, 1 g. daily.
2. After thyroid extract ingestion.
3. Anxiety state. The sleeping BMR is normal.
4. Pyrexia. Increases the BMR.—
   a. 1° F. by + 7 per cent.
   b. 1° C. by + 13 per cent.
5. Congestive cardiac failure—there is excessive action of the respiratory muscles, and the slow circulation-rate leads to excessive oxygen utilization.
6. Leukæmia.—
   a. Acute cases of all types.
   b. Chronic myeloid leukæmia.
7. Polycythæmia vera. A moderate increase frequently occurs.

8. Carcinomatosis.
9. Phæochromocytoma.
10. Increase occurs in some cases of—
    a. Hyperpituitarism.—
        i. Gigantism } In the early stages.
        ii. Acromegaly } In the early stages.
        iii. Cushing's syndrome.
    b. Diabetes insipidus. The BMR is reduced by pitressin therapy.
    c. Hodgkin's disease.
    d. Hyperadrenalism.
    e. Essential hypertension.
    f. Pernicious anæmia, especially in the presence of subacute combined degeneration of the spinal cord.
    g. Hæmochromatosis.
    h. Steatorrhœa.

Decrease.—
1. Hypothyroidism. The BMR may fall to −30 per cent to − 45 per cent. The BMR rises after thyroid extract 1 gr. daily for 10–14 days.
2. Hypopituitarism leading to secondary hypothyroidism.
3. Malnutrition.
4. Nephrosis, with œdema. The BMR is lowest when the œdema is greatest.
5. Severe anæmia.
6. Shock.
7. Prolonged rest in bed.
8. Depressive psychoses.
9. Drugs.—
    a. Thiouracil and other similar drugs.
    b. Morphine.
    c. Chloral hydrate.
    d. Barbiturates and other sedatives and hypnotics.
10. Addison's disease (some cases).
11. Hypogonadism (some cases).

N.B.—**Where facilities are available, estimation of radioactive iodine uptake by the thyroid gland is more accurate than estimation of the BMR.**

REFERENCES.—Aub, J. C., and Du Bois, E. F. (1917), *Arch. intern. Med.*, **19**, 823; Robertson, J. D., and Reid, D. D. (1952), *Lancet*, **1**, 940; Crooks, J., Murray, I. P. C., and Wayne, E. J. (1958), *Ibid.*, **1**, 604 (this paper compares Aub's and Du Bois' standards with those of Robertson and Reid).

BENCE JONES PROTEIN IN URINE

This is an abnormal protein which precipitates at about 40–50° C., and certainly at less than 60° C. It has a molecular weight of 40,000 and an electrophoretic mobility the same as, or similar to, the associated abnormal serum globulin fraction. The protein consists of light chains in dimers (*see* Immunoglobulins).

Bence Jones protein appears in the urine.—
    Most commonly in:—
        1. Multiple myeloma.

Uncommonly in:—
  2. Osteogenic sarcoma.
  3. Osteomalacia.
  4. Multiple secondary deposits of carcinoma in bone.
  5. Lymphatic and myeloid leukæmia.
  6. Severe empyema.
  7. It may be demonstrated in some renal conditions
     in which there has been long-standing proteinuria.
  8. Occasionally in some cases of pyuria, a substance
     giving a positive reaction on heating may be found.
     A similar reaction may be given by urine con-
     taminated with seminal vesicle fluid.
  9. Polycythæmia vera.
 10. Macroglobulinæmia.

REFERENCE.—Porter, R. R. (1963), *Brit. med. Bull.*, **19**, 197.

STANDARD BICARBONATE IN BLOOD

This is the concentration of bicarbonate in whole blood at
38° C. equilibrated at a Pco_2 of 40 mm. Hg with the blood
hæmoglobin fully oxygenated.

Normal Range.—21·3–24·8 mEq./litre (mean = 23 mEq./litre).
(21·3–24·8 mmol./litre.)

Other Estimations.—
  1. *Plasma Bicarbonate.*—The concentration of bicarbonate
     in plasma, plus small amounts of carbonate and carb-
     amino compounds.
  2. *Plasma Carbon Dioxide Content,* or *Total Carbon Dioxide
     Concentration.*—The carbon dioxide extractable from
     plasma by strong acid, which includes bicarbonate,
     dissolved carbon dioxide, carbonic acid, carbonate, and
     carbamino compounds.
        Normal range—23–33 mEq./litre (53–75 vol. per cent).
        Mean value—28 mEq./litre (62 vol. per cent).
  3. *Plasma Alkali Reserve (Plasma Carbon Dioxide Capacity).*—
     The plasma carbon dioxide content after equilibration of
     the plasma at Pco_2 of 40 mm. Hg.
  4. *Arterial Bicarbonate.*—This is the plasma CO_2 content
     minus $(0.03 \times Pco_2)$, i.e., approximately 1 mEq./litre less
     than the equivalent plasma CO_2 content.
  5. *Carbonic Acid Content of Plasma.—*
        (Pco_2 in mm. Hg $\times 0.03$) mmol./litre.
  6. *Partial Pressure of Carbon Dioxide in Plasma* (Pco_2).—
     That pressure which is exerted by carbon dioxide present
     in physical solution, and which is proportional to its
     concentration in solution. In arterial blood it is equal to
     the pressure exerted by carbon dioxide in alveolar air
     (40 mm. Hg). As Pco_2 increases, the rate and depth
     of respiration increase, and vice versa, due to direct action
     on the medullary respiratory centre. Above a concentration
     of 9 per cent carbon dioxide acts as a depressant. As
     Pco_2 increases, more carbonic acid is formed, and vice
     versa.
        Normal pulmonary ventilation rate—5–7 litres/min.

Increase CO_2 concentration by 0·3 per cent—ventilation rate is doubled.

At CO_2 concentration of 9 per cent—ventilation rate is 50–70 litres/min.

Physiology.—

The enzyme carbonic anhydrase, which is present in red blood-cells and the distal renal tubules, gastric mucosa, etc., catalyses the reaction:—

$$H_2O + CO_2 \rightleftharpoons H_2CO_3$$

Carbonic acid ionizes slightly:—

$$H_2CO_3 \rightleftharpoons H^+ + HCO_3^-$$

Bicarbonate salts ionize much more completely:—

$$BHCO_3 \rightleftharpoons B^+ + HCO_3^-$$

The ratio of $BHCO_3$ (or HCO_3) to un-ionized H_2CO_3 is normally about 20 to 1 in normal plasma. From the Henderson-Hasselbalch equation,

$$\text{plasma } pH = pK + \log \cdot \frac{[BHCO_3]}{[H_2CO_3]} = 6\cdot1 + 1\cdot3 = 7\cdot4$$

(where pK is the dissociation constant).

Thus, the plasma pH is determined by this ratio of bicarbonate/carbonic acid. The bicarbonate concentration can be varied, increasing with anion deficit, decreasing with cation deficit, to maintain cation/anion balance in the extracellular fluid. After a relative or absolute increase in anions, bicarbonate in plasma falls with loss of carbon dioxide and water in the lungs. If, on the other hand, anions decrease relative to cations, more bicarbonate rapidly forms.

When plasma pH rises, respiration is depressed and shallow, and when plasma pH falls, respiration is stimulated (below pH 7·0 it is no longer effective). After any change in anion/cation balance the plasma pH is kept within the normal range by the maintenance of the bicarbonate/carbonic acid ratio (until the anion/cation disturbance is gross). By variation in the rate of respiration (regulated in its turn by small changes in plasma Pco_2 and plasma pH), and by variation in renal bicarbonate excretion, the plasma alkali reserve is kept within normal limits. (A change in plasma pH of less than 0·1 has an effect on the respiration rate. When the plasma pH falls by 0·2 to 7·2 the ventilation rate rises to 35 litres per min.)

Pathological.—

Increased Standard Bicarbonate.—

1. *Respiratory Acidosis.*—Following excessive CO_2 retention, more carbonic acid forms. To maintain the normal plasma pH, the bicarbonate fraction also increases. Thus the alkali reserve in plasma is abnormally raised in:—

    a. Poor exchange of gases between alveolar air and plasma, and between alveolar air and external air, in:—
        i. Emphysema.
        ii. Pneumonia.
        iii. Cardiac failure with pulmonary congestion.
        iv. Progressive lung destruction.

    b. Depression of the respiratory centre:—
        i. Due to the action of morphine.

ii. During anæsthesia.

Since Pco$_2$ increases, H$_2$CO$_3$ increases relatively more than BHCO$_3$. Thus in decompensation the ratio of bicarbonate/carbonic acid falls, and the plasma pH falls.

2. *Metabolic Alkalosis.*—Following excessive intake of cation (e.g., sodium as bicarbonate, lactate or citrate) the bicarbonate fraction increases to balance the excess cation. To maintain the normal bicarbonate/carbonic acid ratio carbon dioxide is retained, but to a relatively smaller degree. Hence, the ratio tends to increase in decompensation, and the plasma pH tends to rise above normal.

   a. Excessive alkali ingestion, e.g., sodium bicarbonate.

   b. Excessive loss of chloride relative to sodium, with resulting increase in sodium/chloride ratio in the extracellular fluid, e.g., persistent vomiting, or continuous gastric aspiration.

   c. Potassium depletion. Sodium and hydrogen ions enter the cells in exchange for potassium ions, resulting in intracellular acidosis and extracellular alkalosis.

Decreased Standard Bicarbonate.—

3. *Respiratory Alkalosis.*—When there is excessive respiratory loss of CO$_2$ via the alveoli, the formation of carbonic acid is depressed. There is an associated fall in the bicarbonate fraction. Since loss of carbon dioxide is relatively greater than bicarbonate retention, it follows that in decompensation the plasma pH tends to rise.

   Overventilation.—

   a. May be voluntary.

   b. May be hysterical.

   c. May occur in cerebral injury.

   d. May occur in heat stroke.

   e. May occur during anæsthesia.

   f. May occur in fever.

N.B.—**Salicylates, and also oxygen lack, stimulate the respiratory centre.**

4. *Metabolic Acidosis.*—Following excessive loss of cation relative to anion, or following excessive formation of organic acids, the rate of ionization of bicarbonate is depressed relatively more than the rate of formation of carbonic acid. Hence the ratio of bicarbonate/carbonic acid falls and the blood pH tends to fall. The falling plasma pH stimulates respiration so that more CO$_2$ is lost from the blood, and the condition is ameliorated:—

   a. Diabetes mellitus. Formation of excess organic acids.

   b. Renal failure. Retention of phosphate and sulphate by the renal tubules.

   c. Ureters transplanted into colon. If the colon is not emptied of urine frequently, excess chloride is reabsorbed.

   d. Starvation. Excess organic acid formation occurs during body-fat breakdown, after the body carbohydrate stores have been used.

   e. Ammonium chloride ingestion. The ammonium group is metabolized by the liver, leaving excess chloride and hydrogen ions in the extracellular fluid. Calcium chloride ingestion also causes metabolic acidosis.

f. Renal tubular acidosis.

g. Severe diarrhœa (relatively a greater loss of sodium than chloride).

REFERENCES.—Harrison, G. A. (1957), *Chemical Methods in Clinical Medicine*, 4th ed. London: Churchill; Morgan, H. G. (1969), *Brit. J. Anæsth.*, **41**, 196.

BICARBONATE IN GASTRIC JUICE

Normal Concentration.—

1. Parietal juice.—Nil.
2. Non-parietal juice.—45 mEq./litre.

BILE-PIGMENTS

BILE-PIGMENTS IN AMNIOTIC FLUID.—Abnormal increase in liquor bilirubin occurs in hæmolytic disease of the newborn, and detection of such an increase has been used as a guide to treatment.

REFERENCE.—Walker, W. (1970), *Brit. med. J.*, **2**, 220.

BILE-PIGMENTS IN FÆCES.—
Normal.—

1. In the newborn, bilirubin colours the stools yellow.
2. With the development of a normal fæcal flora of bacteria, bilirubin is converted to stercobilin, and the adult brown colour of normal fæces develops. When intestinal hurry occurs in an infant, incomplete oxidation may occur and biliverdin colours the fæces green.
3. In the normal adult, little or no bilirubin appears in the stools.

Pathological.—

1. In severe diarrhœa, a little bilirubin may be present.
2. After some antibiotics, e.g., aureomycin, the formation of stercobilin is inhibited, and bilirubin appears in the fæces.
3. *Absence of Pigment (Stercobilin) in Stool.—*
   a. Obstruction to the flow of bile.
   b. Suppression of bile formation.

For an account of other pigments in fæces in disease, and particularly after drugs or change in diet, see *Chemical Methods in Clinical Medicine* by Harrison.

REFERENCE.—Harrison, G. A. (1957), *Chemical Methods in Clinical Medicine*, 4th ed. London : Churchill.

BILE-PIGMENTS IN URINE.—
Normal.—Bilirubin is not detected in the urine by routine methods, e.g., Fouchet's test.

1. Free bilirubin (unconjugated) is probably not excreted by the kidney in the absence of renal damage.
2. The renal threshold for conjugated bilirubin (conjugated with glycuronate) is low. Thus, in the pre-icteric stage of acute hepatitis bilirubin appears in the urine. Bilirubin diglycuronate is more rapidly excreted than bilirubin monoglycuronate.

Pathological (i.e., qualitative routine tests for bilirubin positive).—

1. Obstructive jaundice.
2. Hepatocellular damage.

N.B.—**Qualitative tests for bilirubin in urine are satisfactory for clinical purposes.**

REFERENCE.—Varley, H. (1954), *Practical Clinical Biochemistry.* London : Heinemann.

BILE-SALTS IN URINE.—Normally 5–10 g. of sodium glycocholate and sodium taurocholate are excreted in the bile each day, assisting in fat absorption and being reabsorbed with fat in the intestine.

Using a crude test (e.g., Hay's "flowers of sulphur" test, bile-salts, although normally present in the urine in low concentration, cannot be detected).

Pathological.—

Hay's Test Positive.—

1. Obstructive jaundice ⎫
2. Acute hepatitis ⎭ In the early stages only.

N.B.—**The presence of traces of detergents, or moderate amounts of protein in the urine, will produce a false-positive test. The test is of little value.**

BILIRUBIN IN SERUM.—
Normal Range.—

At birth—0·4–4·0 mg./100 ml.
3 days—1·0–10·0 mg./100 ml.
1 month—0·3–1·0 mg./100 ml.
Adult—0·1–0·5 mg./100 ml. (2–9 mmol./litre).

$$\left(\frac{\text{mg./litre}}{585} = \mu\text{mol./litre.} \right)$$

Physiology.—200–370 mg. of bilirubin are excreted in the bile each day, derived from 7–8 g. of hæmoglobin. Passage through the liver cells of free bilirubin, derived from the breakdown of hæmoglobin, results in its conjugation with glycuronic acid.

The van den Bergh "direct" reaction is given by bilirubin conjugated with glycuronic acid, which is comparatively more soluble in water. Free, unconjugated, bilirubin gives an "indirect" reaction on diazotization, because it is more soluble in organic solvents. The direct/indirect ratio (D.I. Ratio) is a measure of the ratio of these pigments. In man it appears that a fairly constant ratio between conjugated and unconjugated bilirubin is maintained regardless of their total concentration in biliary tract obstruction.

REFERENCE.—Acocella, G., Tenconi, L. T., Armas-Merino, R., Raia, S., and Billing, Barbara, H. (1968), *Lancet*, **1**, 68.

Physiological.—
Increase.—

1. Increases occur in the infant's serum during the first few days after birth.
2. Increases in the serum bilirubin occur in untrained people at high altitudes.

Decrease.—The conjugating enzyme system is induced by phenobarbitone, and epileptics on long-term therapy have lower serum bilirubin levels than normal controls.

Pathological.—

Increase.

1. *Simple Biliary Obstruction.*—Bilirubin diffuses from the hepatic cells, after conjugation with glycuronate, back into the blood-stream. (The van den Bergh reaction is "direct positive". Later, in unrelieved obstruction, liver damage occurs, and the indirect fraction increases.)

2. *Hepatocellular Damage.*—Because the parenchymal liver cells are damaged, conjugation of bilirubin is impaired. (The van den Bergh reaction is "direct negative" and "indirect positive".)

3. *Overproduction of Bilirubin.*—Excessive amounts of bilirubin reach the liver cells. Serum level of unconjugated bilirubin is increased. (The van den Bergh reaction is "direct negative" and "indirect positive".)

4. *Overproduction of Bilirubin, associated with Impaired Liver Function.*—In addition to the increased serum concentration of free bilirubin, some conjugated bilirubin diffuses back into the blood-stream. (The van den Bergh reaction is "direct positive" and "indirect positive".) If serum bilirubin exceeds 5 mg./100 ml. in hæmolytic anæmia, there is probably also hepatic dysfunction.

The diagnosis of biliary obstruction or liver-cell damage by means of the presence or absence of a positive direct van den Bergh reaction, or of hæmolytic jaundice by the presence of an indirect positive, direct negative reaction, is unfortunately an oversimplification. When obstruction persists, the liver cells are damaged, and in most cases involving hepatocellular damage there is some associated intrahepatic biliary obstruction.

Following prednisolone 30 mg. daily for 5 days the serum bilirubin falls by more than 40 per cent in hepatocellular jaundice but is unchanged in jaundice due to cholestasis. There is no increase in red-cell life, no significant increase in conjugation, and only slight increase in the rate of bile-pigment excretion; probably steroids increase pigment storage in the liver cells. This is a diagnostic and not a therapeutic test and following the high steroid dosage "tailing off" doses of prednisolone should be given during the following 4 weeks.

It is worth noting that after relief of a simple biliary obstruction, the serum alkaline phosphatase concentration falls more slowly towards normal than does the serum bilirubin. At this stage the bilirubin in the serum is predominantly in the unconjugated state (van den Bergh reaction, direct negative), as it is during recovery from hepatitis.

The serial estimation of the serum bilirubin concentration, in conjunction with other tests of liver function, is far more useful in assessing prognosis and diagnosis than is a single estimation of serum bilirubin. A jaundiced patient always has a raised serum bilirubin level, at the onset of jaundice, but not necessarily during recovery.

REFERENCES.—Malloy, H. T., and Evelyn, K. A. (1937), *J. biol. Chem.*, **119**, 481, and (1958), *Brit. med. J.*, **2**, 785 (Annotation on congenital hyperbilirubinæmia); King, E. J., and Coxon, V. J. (1950), *J. clin. Path.*, **3**, 248; Cole, P. G., and Lathe, G. H. (1953), *Ibid.*, **6**, 99 (Separation of the serum pigments).

SERUM BILIRUBIN AND ALKALINE PHOSPHATASE IN LIVER DISEASE (*Fig.* 1).—

By way of generalization, the following patterns in uncomplicated liver disorders are described:—

Progressive increase in abnormal readings indicates deterioration. Progressive return towards normal values implies recovery.

Group 1.—Uncomplicated extrahepatic biliary obstruction, cholangitis, and cholangiolitis.

Group 2.—Diffuse hepatocellular damage. (Also in hæmolytic conditions.)

Group 3.—Portal cirrhosis (some cases), liver abscess, secondary carcinomatosis of the liver, and sarcoidosis involving the liver.

Group 4.—Increasing hepatocellular damage superimposed on bile-duct obstruction.

N.B.—Obstruction of one major bile-duct with a patent common bile-duct leads to an abnormally raised serum alkaline phosphatase level with normal serum bilirubin levels, i.e., more liver substance may be needed to excrete alkaline phosphatase than bilirubin in the bile.

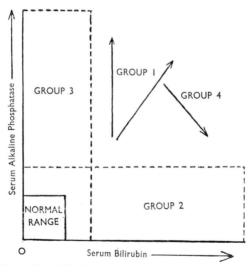

Fig. 1.—Serum bilirubin and alkaline phosphatase in liver disease.

OCCULT BLOOD IN FÆCES

Daily blood-loss into the intestinal tract, and hence the stools, is up to 2·5 ml./day in normal subjects.

Guiac tests become positive after 10 ml. or more of blood are shed into the gastro-intestinal tract, whilst the phenolphthalein test is positive after 3·5–20 ml. of blood, and the orthotolidine test is positive after 1–25 ml. of blood are shed.

Obviously the tests are affected by the diet, the rate of intestinal passage of contents, and the presence of interfering or enhancing substances.

False-positive occult-blood test results are obtained with plant and bacterial peroxidases, fresh bleeding from lesions in the lower intestinal tract, or blood in the diet (e.g., black pudding, etc.). Iron salts affect some methods.

The withdrawal of benzidine from test systems has resulted in a reappraisal of this test, since the various methods can be adjusted to give positive results at different degrees of bloodloss—the test is not simply indicating the absolute presence or absence of bleeding in the gut, and a decision has to be made as to the degree of sensitivity of the test which is useful to the clinician.

REFERENCE.—Editorial (1970), *Lancet*, **1**, 819.

BROMSULPHTHALEIN IN SERUM

Test.—5 mg. of dye per kg. body-weight are injected intravenously in the form of a 5 per cent aqueous solution. This is assumed to produce a maximum serum concentration of 10 mg./100 ml. Blood samples are usually taken at 25 minutes and 45 minutes after injection, for dye estimation.

Normal.—
1. Less than 25 per cent of the dye remains in the 15-minute sample.
2. Less than 15 per cent of the dye remains in the 25-minute sample.
3. Less than 5 per cent of the dye remains in the 45-minute sample.

(The 15-minute and 25-minute samples are not essential.)

The mechanism of excretion of the dye is similar to that of bilirubin, but the load on the liver is much greater. Therefore, in all cases of jaundice other than those due to excessive red blood-cell hæmolysis, the rate of removal will be reduced, and the performance of the test would therefore be pointless. Œstrogens impair the disposal of bromsulphthalein by the normal liver.

This test is a most sensitive and specific measure of hepatic function. The normal elderly subject shows moderate impairment. The major metabolic pathway in man, rat, dog, and other species involves the conjugation of the dye with glutathione, catalysed by a non-specific glutathione-conjugating enzyme. Impaired conjugation can be due to:—
1. Depression of enzyme activity.
2. Low hepatic glutathione levels.

Pathological.—
Increased Removal of the Dye.—The rate of elimination is increased via the urine in cases with albuminuria. This may mask faulty elimination by a damaged liver.

Decreased Removal of the Dye.—

1. *Liver Disease.*—Any type of generalized liver disease, for example:—
    a. Advanced cirrhosis of the liver.
    b. Chronic hepatitis.
    c. All types of jaundice other than hæmolytic jaundice.
    d. Congestive cardiac failure, with venous congestion of the liver. (Recovery from failure can be demonstrated by diminished dye retention.)
    N.B.—In the presence of ascites the dye passes into the ascitic fluid and is bound to albumin. Thus an appreciable amount is lost from the plasma without any liver activity. Bromsulphthalein, injected intraperitoneally, can be used to measure the volume of ascitic fluid.
    e. Following portacaval anastomosis.
    f. Following repeated halothane exposure.
2. *Gall-bladder Disease.*—
    a. Acute cholecystitis.
    b. Chronic cholecystitis (only in acute exacerbation).
    c. Morphine administration. This causes spasm of the bile-duct sphincter, with abnormal retention.
3. Rarely, excessive reabsorption from the bowel has occurred after excretion in the bile.
4. Œstrogens impair metabolism of bromsulphthalein by the normal liver.

N.B.—

1. After meals the rate of excretion is greatly increased, due to increased hepatic blood-flow and bile secretion. The test should therefore be performed fasting.
2. The dye is an irritant. There should be no leak around the vein at injection.

REFERENCES.—Burnett, W. (1954), *Lancet*, **1**, 488 (The effect of cholecystitis); Thompson, E. N., Sherlock, S., and Williams, R. (1964), *Lancet*, **2**, 1352; Biebuyck, J. F., Saunders, S. J., Harrison, G. G., and Bull, A. B. (1970), *Brit. med. J.*, **1**, 669.

BUFFER BASE IN BLOOD

The buffer base of blood is the sum of the buffer anions, and includes bicarbonate in plasma and red cells, plasma proteins, phosphates, hæmoglobin, and oxyhæmoglobin.

Normal Range.—45–50 mEq./litre (mean=47·5 mEq./litre).
The value varies with the hæmoglobin content.—
Normal buffer base at pH 7·38 and P_{CO_2} 40 mm. Hg,

$$= 40·8 + 0·36 \times (\text{Hb in g./100 ml.})$$

or

$$= 41·7 + 0·42 \times (\text{Hb in g./100 ml.}).$$

Base Excess.—This represents the base concentration of whole blood on titration with strong acid to pH 7·4 at a P_{CO_2} of 40 mm. Hg at 37° C., and normal values are within the range of $-2·3-+2·3$ mEq./litre (mean=0).

Base excess = Blood buffer base − normal buffer base.

Pathological.—
  Base Deficit (or negative base excess).—
  1. After acute myocardial infarction.
  2. Cyanotic congenital heart disease.
  3. Chronic renal disease.
  4. Diabetic ketosis.

CALCITONIN IN PLASMA

Normal calcitonin is formed in the parafollicular cells in the thyroid and inhibits bone resorption, i.e., a physiological antagonist to parathyroid hormone, blocking calcium mobilization by the latter from bone. Output of calcitonin is increased by hypercalcæmia, and suppressed by hypocalcæmia. It has a half-life of 4–15 minutes and the normal plasma level= 0–12 ng./ml. Estimation of this polypeptide has proved to be difficult so far.

Pathological.—
  Increase.—
  1. Pseudohypoparathyroidism.
  2. Medullary carcinoma of the thyroid.
  3. ? In osteopetrosis.
  Decrease.—
  1. Hyperparathyroidism.
  2. Gorlin's syndrome.

REFERENCES.—Foster, G. V. (1968), *Postgrad. med. J.*, **44**, 411; Clark, M. B., Boyd, G. W., Byfield, P. G. H., and Foster, G. V. (1969), *Lancet*, **2**, 74; Gadmundson, T. V., Galante, L., Woodhouse, N. J. Y., Matthews, E. W., Osato, T. D., MacIntyre, I., Kenny, A. D., and Wiggins, R. C. (1969), *Ibid.*, **1**, 443.

CALCIUM

CALCIUM INFUSION TEST.—Intravenous infusion of 15 mg. of calcium per kg. body-weight is given over a period of 4 hours, in the form of calcium gluconate solution.

Results.—
  1. In simple osteomalacia and in some cases of steatorrhœa before the development of other evidence of osteomalacia, the increase in the 0–12-hour urine calcium excretion is low.
  2. By measuring the 4-hour serum calcium rise and the 4-hour excess urine calcium loss, it is possible to measure the calcium deposited in the bone. This deposition is defective in osteoporosis.
  3. The serum inorganic phosphate rises and the urine phosphate falls in normal individuals, maximally at 8–12 hours. These changes are excessive in secondary hyperparathyroidism (osteomalacia). They are minimal in primary hyperparathyroidism, vitamin-D poisoning, and primary renal tubular disease.

REFERENCES.—Nordin, B. E. C., and Fraser, R. (1954), *Clin. Sci.*, **13**, 477 (1956), *Lancet*, **1**, 823.

CALCIUM IN CEREBROSPINAL FLUID.—Normally the calcium present in the cerebrospinal fluid is in the ionized form. The normal range is 5·5–6·00 mg./100 ml. (2·75–3·0 mEq./litre)

The concentration is identical with the ionized fraction present in the serum. A cerebrospinal fluid calcium of less than 6 mg./ 100 ml. in the presence of hypercalcæmia suggests primary hyper-parathyroidism. The cerebrospinal fluid does not reflect serum calcium changes of hypoparathyroidism.

The total cerebrospinal fluid calcium increases and un-ionized calcium appears in conditions in which the cerebrospinal fluid protein is increased.

REFERENCE.—Howard, J. E., Carey, R. A., Rubin, P. S., and Levine, M. D. (1949), *Trans. Ass. Amer. Physns*, **62**, 264.

CALCIUM IN FÆCES.—
Normal Output.—On an average diet: < 560 mg./24 hr.
The daily output varies with the diet.

Increase.—
1. Vitamin-D deficiency.
2. High phytic acid content in diet, e.g., oatmeal. Calcium phytate is insoluble.
3. High phosphate diet.
4. Many cases of nephrosis.
5. Steatorrhœa and malabsorption syndromes.
   In these conditions, the fæcal calcium is high because the dietary calcium is not being absorbed.

Decrease.—
1. Osteomalacia successfully treated with vitamin D.
2. Hypervitaminosis D.
   In these latter two conditions, more calcium is absorbed from the diet than normal.
3. Low phosphate content in diet.
4. Some cases of Boeck's sarcoid. Increased calcium absorption from diet can be reduced by cortisone.

N.B.—**Fæcal calcium estimations are only useful as part of metabolic balance studies.**

REFERENCE.—Varley, H. (1954), *Practical Clinical Biochemistry*. London : Heinemann.

CALCIUM IN SERUM.—
Normal Range.—
Normal males.—9·04–10·30 mg./100 ml.
   At 20 years = 9·09–10·20 mg./100 ml.
   At 70 years = 8·77–9·88 mg./100 ml.
Normal females.—8·93–10·05 mg./100 ml.
   No change with age.

Using EDTA titration methods the normal range = 8·5–10·5 mg./100 ml. (4·3–5·3 mEq./litre; 2·2–2·6 mmol./litre).

$$\left(\frac{\text{mg./litre}}{40} = \text{mmol./litre.}\right)$$

(Results by atomic absorption method are approximately +0·2 mg./100 ml. above equivalent results by EDTA titration methods.)

REFERENCE.—Yendt, E. R., and Gagne, R. J. A. (1968), *Can. med. Ass. J.*, **98**, 331.

N.B.—**Calcium is present in tap water, and calcium soaps adhere to glass. Therefore always use carefully prepared syringes, containers, and glassware for blood collection for this test.**

Physiological.—

 Increase.—Within the normal range, the serum level is higher in summer than in winter.

 Decrease.—Within the normal range, the serum level falls after increased carbohydrate utilization, or after insulin administration. Normal meals can produce an increase in serum calcium of over 1 mg./100 ml. Therefore fasting blood samples should always be examined.

Pathological.—

 Increase.—

1. Hyperparathyroidism. If this diagnosis is considered and a normal blood-level is obtained, repeat the estimation at weekly intervals, as the blood level fluctuates. Also estimate the daily urine calcium excretion, which is increased. The plasma inorganic phosphate concentration should be estimated at the same time. The serum level is unaffected by cortisone therapy.
2. Hypervitaminosis D (especially with added calcium in the diet). Hypercalcæmia corrected by steroids.
3. Multiple myelomatosis (some cases).
4. Multiple carcinomatous bone secondary deposits (some cases). Urine calcium excretion is increased in most cases. If cortisone inhibits neoplastic growth, it will also cause a fall in a raised serum calcium level.
5. Acute bone atrophy (especially in children with fractures or poliomyelitis and immobilization).
6. Renal disease (very rare). The level is usually low.
7. Excessive alkali intake (peptic ulcer cases), if the antacid contains calcium, or if milk is taken in excess.
8. Prolonged respiratory alkalæmia.
9. Boeck's sarcoid (some cases). Hypercalcæmia corrected by steroids.
10. Acromegaly (some cases).
11. Cushing's syndrome (some cases with osteoporosis).
12. Paget's disease with pathological fracture and subsequent immobilization.
13. Polycythæmia vera (slight rise, cause unknown).
14. Idiopathic hypercalcæmia. Oral calcium load test results in sustained hypercalcæmia.

 Decrease.—

1. Hypoparathyroidism.
2. Pseudohypoparathyroidism.
3. Vitamin-D deficiency.
4. Steatorrhœa (faulty absorption of vitamin D, calcium, and phosphorus).
5. Nephrosis. The non-ionized fraction carried by the serum protein is affected, probably being lost in the urine.
6. Renal disease with phosphate retention.
7. Acute pancreatitis. The fatty acids liberated by the action of pancreatic lipase bind calcium. In hæmorrhagic pancreatitis serum calcium falls by the third day. The serum calcium does not fall in the œdematous form.

8. Intravenous magnesium salts, oxalates, or citrates.
9. In senile osteoporosis the serum calcium level may be at the lower limit of the normal range.
10. Neonatal hypocalcæmia.
    a. First day.—
        i. Low birth-weight.
        ii. Maternal diabetes mellitus.
        iii. Maternal placenta prævia.
        iv. Maternal toxæmia.
    b. Fifth to tenth days.—Associated with hyperphosphatæmia induced in some infants by cow's milk.
11. Plasma ionized calcium is reduced in hypomagnesæmia. ? Cause of tetany.

N.B.—
1. Tetany may occur if the serum total calcium falls below 6–7 mg./100 ml. (3–3·5 mEq./litre).
2. Tetany occurs with normal serum calcium levels in both metabolic and respiratory alkalæmia.
3. If the plasma potassium concentration is abnormally low, then the serum calcium level may fall to lower levels before tetany develops.   But tetany may occur at low potassium values when the serum calcium is normal if the intracellular sodium and potassium concentrations are high. (*See* section on Potassium.)
4. Ultrafilterable fraction corresponds roughly with the ionized fraction. "Ionized calcium" may be roughly calculated as:—

$$6·5 \times \frac{\text{total serum calcium mg. } \% + 0·7}{\text{total serum protein g. } \% + 6·6} - 0·65.$$

5. Where total calcium increases in disease, after calcium infusion, or after parathormone administration, both free and bound calcium rise in proportion.
6. In hypocalcæmia, the ultrafilterable fraction is normal or raised when expressed as a percentage of the total calcium. Approximately 0·8 mg. calcium is bound by 1 g. of protein.
7. Spurious hypocalcæmia is found when blood from renal patients on maintenance dialysis is stored before estimation.

REFERENCES.—Clark, E. P., and Collip, J. B. (1925), *J. biol. Chem.*, **63**, 461; Terepka, A. R., Toribara, T. Y., and Dewey, P. A. (1958), *J. clin. Invest.*, **37**, 87; Barr, D. G. D., and Forfar, J. D. (1963), *Brit. med. J.*, **1**, 477; Winstone, N. E. (1965), *Brit. J. Surg.*, **52**, 804; Oppé, T. E., and Redstone, D. (1968), *Lancet*, **1**, 1045; Coburn, J., Massry, S. G., Gordon, Sybil, and Rubin, M. E. (1969), *Amer. J. Clin. Path.*, **52**, 572.

CALCIUM IN URINE.—On a normal diet the normal daily output of calcium in the urine is 100–300 mg./24 hr. (50–150 mEq./24 hr.).

On a dietary intake of less than 200 mg./24 hr. urine calcium output = 13–180 mg./24 hr.

On a dietary intake of 200–600 mg./24 hr. urine calcium output = 50–200 mg./24 hr.

On a dietary intake of approx. 1 g./24 hr. urine calcium output = <300 mg./24 hr.

In the absence of avitaminosis D, the renal threshold for calcium is approximately 7 mg./100 ml. (3·5 mEq./litre).

Urine output of calcium falls in late normal pregnancy.

REFERENCE.—Hodgkinson, A., and Pyrah, L. N. (1958), *Brit. J. Surg.*, **46**, 10.

Increased Output.—

1. Hyperparathyroidism. More than 300 mg./24 hr. is suspicious, if a normal diet is being eaten. About one-third of all cases may have a normal urine calcium output.
2. Osteolytic bone metastases (carcinoma and sarcoma).
3. Myeloma.
4. Osteoporosis.—
   a. Especially after immobilization.
   b. Cushing's syndrome.
   c. Acromegaly.
   d. Following large doses of corticosteroid drugs.
5. Vitamin-D intoxication. Hypercalcuria occurs in many cases before the serum calcium rises.
6. Sarcoidosis (some cases).
7. Renal tubule acidosis.—The tubules do not form either ammonia or hydrogen ions. Therefore there is excessive loss of base.
8. Idiopathic hypercalcuria.—Possibly this condition is due to diminished renal tubular reabsorption of calcium. Fifty per cent of cases excrete more than 300 mg./24 hr. whilst on a normal diet.
9. Thyrotoxicosis.—X-rays show rarefaction of the skeleton in many cases.
10. Paget's disease.
11. Fanconi's syndrome.
12. Hepatolenticular degeneration.
13. Frusemide therapy.
14. Stone-formers and relatives of stone-formers excrete more calcium than controls after sugar ingestion.

Decreased Output.—

1. All cases in which the serum calcium is low, other than renal disease.
2. Long-standing milk and alkali diet. In this case the serum calcium is increased when renal failure supervenes.
3. Many cases of nephrosis.
4. Acute nephritis, partly due to decreased intestinal absorption.
5. Benzothiadiazine diuretics.

N.B.—**The Sulkowitch Test for urine calcium is useful as a rapid screening test.**

REFERENCES.—Shohl, A. T., and Pedley, F. G. (1922), *J. biol. Chem.*, **50**, 537; Barney, J. D., and Sulkowitch, H. W. (1937), *J. Urol.*, **37**, 751; Nordin, B. E. C. (1959), *Lancet*, **2**, 368; Lemarr, J., jun., Piering, W. F., and Lennon, E. J. (1969), *New Engl. J. Med.*, **280**, 232.

CARBON DIOXIDE IN BLOOD
(*ARTERIAL* P_{CO_2})

Arterial P_{CO_2} is the partial pressure exerted in arterial blood by dissolved carbon dioxide. Air in the alveoli is normally separated from the blood in the pulmonary capillaries by 0.3–$0.7\ \mu$. This separation may increase in disease. The diffusing capacity of carbon dioxide is about twenty-five times that of oxygen, accounting for differences in response to changes in ventilation in disease between P_{CO_2} and P_{O_2}.

Normal Range.—36–44 mm. Hg pressure. This is the partial pressure exerted by carbon dioxide at the alveolar interface. If the Basal Metabolic Rate is kept constant the partial pressure exerted by carbon dioxide is inversely proportional to the alveolar ventilation. A normal adult produces about 15,000 mEq./day of carbon dioxide.

Pathological.—

1. *Respiratory Acidosis.*—P_{CO_2} tends to rise above normal range as the blood pH tends to fall and the plasma bicarbonate increases.
   In mild hypercapnia the P_{CO_2} rises to 44–88 mm. Hg, and this level is tolerable for short periods. A P_{CO_2} of 80–200 mm. Hg induces narcosis. Levels above 200 mm. Hg are dangerous even for short periods.

2. *Respiratory Alkalosis.*—P_{CO_2} tends to fall below normal range as the blood pH tends to rise and the plasma bicarbonate falls.

3. *Metabolic Acidosis.*—P_{CO_2} tends to fall below normal range as the blood pH tends to fall and the plasma bicarbonate falls.

4. *Metabolic Alkalosis.*—P_{CO_2} tends to rise above normal range as the blood pH tends to rise and the plasma bicarbonate rises.

5. *Hypothermia.*—P_{CO_2} falls as the blood pH and bicarbonate rise with falling body temperature.

Since the P_{CO_2} value can be calculated from the blood pH and plasma bicarbonate concentration, the greatest use for its estimation is in cases of mixed pathology, e.g., salicylate poisoning results in both metabolic acidosis and also respiratory alkalosis from stimulation of the respiratory centre. Knowledge of the P_{CO_2} value is a valuable guide to treatment in cases of pulmonary disease with respiratory distress. It is also very useful when heart–lung machines are used, and when hypothermia is used.

REFERENCE.—Astrup, P., Jorgensen, K., Andersen, O. S., and Engel, K. (1960), *Lancet*, 1, 1035.

CARBOXYHÆMOGLOBIN IN BLOOD

Hæmoglobin has a greater affinity for carbon monoxide than oxygen. The higher the carboxyhæmoglobin concentration in the blood, the less hæmoglobin will be available for oxygen carriage. Therefore anæmic patients will suffer from carbon monoxide poisoning sooner and more severely than normal people. Also, the hæmoglobin oxygen dissociation curve is shifted to the left, and therefore oxygen release to the tissues is less effective. The rate of absorption of carbon monoxide is increased in proportion to the physical activity.

CARBON MONOXIDE IN INSPIRED AIR.—A concentration of:
(1) 0·1 per cent produces a blood carboxyhæmoglobin concentration of about 50 per cent in one hour; (2) 0·2 per cent will cause death within a few hours; (3) 0·4 per cent is fatal in less than one hour; (4) 1 per cent produces a lethal blood concentration in less than 10 minutes. In a fire victim, if the blood carboxyhæmoglobin concentration is 10 per cent or less, death occurred before the fire started.

BLOOD CARBOXYHÆMOGLOBIN CONCENTRATIONS.—

1. Normal tobacco smoker—up to 5 per cent carboxyhæmoglobin.
2. Symptom-free—up to 15–20 per cent carboxyhæmoglobin.
3. Nausea, weakness, and dyspnœa—up to 50 per cent carboxyhæmoglobin.
4. Unconsciousness—50–70 per cent carboxyhæmoglobin.
5. Rapid death—more than 80 per cent carboxyhæmoglobin.

N.B.—

1. Carboxyhæmoglobin can only be detected by using a direct vision spectroscope when the blood concentration exceeds 30 per cent.
2. Rapid accurate estimation of concentrations greater than 5–10 per cent can be made using a reversion spectroscope.
3. Compression in 2 atmospheres of oxygen helps to eliminate carbon monoxide and reduces the damaging period of anoxia. Elimination of 50 per cent of the carbon monoxide in the blood occurs in 2–3 hours of breathing air, and in 15–30 minutes of breathing pure oxygen.

REFERENCE.—Harrison, G. A. (1957), *Chemical Methods in Clinical Medicine*, 4th ed. London : Churchill.

CAROTENOIDS

CAROTENOIDS IN SERUM.—
Normal Range.—100–300 µg./100 ml. consisting of true vitamin A and other carotenoid substances.
Physiological.—
Increase.—
1. Excessively high carrot intake. Oranges also contain carotenoids.
2. Postprandial hyperlipæmia.
Decrease.—Low carotenoid diet. The blood level falls within 1 week of onset of a carotenoid-poor diet, whereas the blood vitamin A is unaffected by dietary change for 6 months, i.e., the body store of carotene is poor, whilst the body stores of vitamin A are large.
Pathological.—
Increase.—
1. Hypothyroidism.
2. Diabetes mellitus.
3. Essential hyperlipæmia, and other forms of hyperlipæmia.
Decrease.—
1. High fever.
2. Liver disease.
3. Malabsorption syndromes, including steatorrhœa.

CAROTENE TOLERANCE TEST.—If the pre-test serum carotene level is low, 20,000 units of beta-carotene in oil are given orally daily for one week.

1. *Normal.*—Serum carotenoids rise to normal by the end of one week.
2. *Malabsorption Syndrome.*—The serum level remains low.

N.B.—Vitamin A is rapidly absorbed from the alimentary tract. Carotene is only slowly absorbed, and on a fat-free diet only 10 per cent of dietary carotene is absorbed. The presence of mineral oils interferes with absorption of carotene.

REFERENCE.—Wenger, J., Kirsner, J. B., and Palmer, W. L. (1957), *Amer. J. Med.*, **22**, 373.

CATECHOLAMINES

CATECHOLAMINES IN BLOOD.—During or shortly after a hypertensive attack caused by a phæochromocytoma the plasma adrenaline-noradrenaline level may rise to 4 µg./100 ml.

Plasma levels of more than 1 µg./100 ml. suggest this cause.

CATECHOLAMINES IN URINE.—

Normal Output.—
1. Noradrenaline—5–100 µg./24 hr.
2. Adrenaline—Average = 11·5 µg./24 hr.

The rate of excretion is greater during the day than during the night. The urine excretion of these amines represents approximately 3 per cent of the total body output.

Pathological.—
1. Essential hypertension. Up to 100 µg./24 hr. may be excreted.
2. Phæochromocytoma. Up to 5000 µg. may be excreted per 24 hours. This increased excretion can be provoked by the administration of histamine.
3. Moderate increase in output:—
   a. After exercise. The normal output after daily routine activity is twice the resting output.
   b. Insulin-induced hypoglycæmia.
   c. Acute coronary artery occlusion.
   d. Severe stress.

N.B.—Bananas contain appreciable amounts of noradrenaline. Therefore remove from diet before collection of urine.

REFERENCE.—Hingerty, D. (1957), *Lancet*, **1**, 766.

Methylated Amines (Metadrenaline+Noradrenaline).—
Normal output = <1 mg./24 hr.; 55 per cent of circulating pressor amines are excreted in this form.
Phæochromocytoma output = 3–113 mg./24 hr.
Increased output in children with neuroblastoma or ganglioneuroma.

REFERENCES.—Pisano, J. J. (1960), *Clin. chim. Acta*, **5**, 406; Brunjes, S., Wynbenga, D., and Johns, V. J., jun. (1964), *Clin. Chem.*, **10**, 1.

4-Hydroxy-3-Methoxy-Mandelic Acid (H.M.M.A. or V.M.A.).—
Normal output = 1·6 µg. per mg. creatinine. (Range = 0·7–2·5 µg.)
Primary hypertension output = 1·5 µg. per mg. creatinine. (Range = 0·5–4·0 µg.)

Phæochromocytoma output=16 μg. per mg. creatinine.
(Range=7·5–30 μg.)

Carcinoid tumour output increased above normal in some cases.
Increased urine output occurs with neuroblastoma and ganglioneuroma in children.

REFERENCES.—Gitlow, S. E., Ornstein, L., Mendlowitz, M., Khassis, S.,
and Kruk, E. (1960), *Amer. J. Med.*, **28**, 921; von Studnitz, W., Käse,
H., and Sjoerdsma, A. (1963), *New Eng. J. Med.*, **269**, 232; Editorial
(1964), *Brit. med. J.*, **1**, 8.

Note.—Methylated amines appear useful in quiescent phases,
free amines are most increased in active phases, in phæochromocytoma. VMA is least increased at any time. Output
is greatly reduced by renal damage.

CEPHALIN CHOLESTEROL IN SERUM

On dilution, serum with an abnormally high globulin content
flocculates with a cephalin-cholesterol mixture. Serum albumin
inhibits the reaction.

Normal Range.—From 0 to + +.

Pathologically Increased Flocculation.—
1. Acute hepatitis. The test is positive before jaundice
   appears, and also before the serum thymol turbidity
   reaction has become positive.
2. Acute hepatic necrosis.
3. Hepatocellular damage, e.g., cirrhosis of the liver.

N.B.—The results obtained with this test are roughly
parallel with those obtained using the thymol turbidity test.
The reagent is not easy to prepare or standardize.

REFERENCES.—Hanger, F. M., and Patek, A. J. (1941), *Amer. J. med.
Sci.*, **202**, 48; Moore, D. B., Pierson, P. S., Hanger, F. M., and Moor,
D. H. (1945), *J. clin. Invest.*, **24**, 292.

CHLORIDE

CHLORIDE IN CEREBROSPINAL FLUID.—

Normal Range.—

Infants.—650–760 mg./100 ml. as sodium chloride.
111–130 mEq./litre as chloride.

Adults.— 700–760 mg./100 ml. as sodium chloride.
120–130 mEq./litre as chloride.

Pathological.—

Increase.—Any condition which causes a rise in the plasma
chloride concentration will cause a proportional rise in the
cerebrospinal chloride.

Decrease.—
1. Any condition which causes a fall in the plasma chloride
   concentration will cause a proportional fall in the
   cerebrospinal chloride.
2. *Meningitis.*—In purulent meningitis, e.g., meningococcal
   meningitis, and especially in tuberculous meningitis, the
   cerebrospinal chloride concentration falls. This fall may
   be due mainly to the associated fall in the plasma level
   following vomiting, but may also be associated with
   alteration in the plasma/cerebrospinal fluid barrier.

REFERENCE.—Doxiadis, S. A., Goldfinch, M. K., and Philpott, M. G.
(1954), *Brit. med. J.*, **1**, 1406.

CHLORIDE IN FÆCES.—The normal daily output of chloride is about 70 mg. as chloride (2 mEq. as chloride).

During moderate diarrhœa the output may increase to 60 mEq. (as chloride) per day. In very severe diarrhœa the fæcal composition approaches that of ileal fluid, and up to 500 mEq. of chloride can be lost in 24 hours.

CHLORIDE IN GASTRIC JUICE.—

Normal Concentration.—
1. Parietal juice.—170 mEq./litre (mmol./litre).
2. Non-parietal juice.—125 mEq./litre (mmol./litre).

CHLORIDE IN PLASMA.—

Normal Range.—
95–105 mEq./litre, as chloride (95–105 mmol./litre).
Males:—
Mean = 101·4 mEq./litre (mmol./litre).
Range = 97–106 mEq./litre (mmol./litre).
Females:—
Mean = 102·4 mEq./litre (mmol./litre).
Range = 98–107 mEq./litre (mmol./litre).

REFERENCE.—Flynn, F. V. (1969), *Ann. Clin. Biochem.*, 6, 1.

Increase.—Similar causes to those provoking hypernatræmia:—
1. Dehydration, after 36–48 hours' duration (12–24 hours in infants).
2. Excess saline parenterally in diabetic ketosis.
3. Excess saline parenterally in advanced renal disease, and also in recovery from acute renal failure. Although the kidneys may eliminate excess sodium ions, the excess chloride ions are not completely eliminated, resulting in hyperchloræmic acidosis. This is because "normal" saline contains excess chloride ions to sodium ions, when compared with the extracellular fluid. The renal tubular ammonium production and hydrogen ion exchange mechanism is impaired.
4. Hyperchloræmic acidosis.—
   a. Lightwood type.
   b. Albright type.
5. Following head injury, associated with hypothalamic stimulation or damage.
6. Excess DOCA or steroid therapy.
7. Relatively greater loss of sodium than chloride, as in severe diarrhœa or intestinal fistula.
8. Excessive reabsorption of chloride by the large bowel, after ureterocolic anastomosis.
9. Respiratory alkalosis.
10. Ion exchange resin therapy to produce a low sodium diet.
11. Acetazolamide therapy. During the diuresis promoted by this substance, sodium, potassium, and bicarbonate ions are lost in the urine.
12. Primary hyperparathyroidism—plasma chloride greater than 102 mEq./litre, whilst in hypercalcæmia due to other causes plasma chloride is less than 102 mEq./litre.

Decrease.—Similar causes to those provoking hyponatræmia:—

1. Low salt diet.
2. Gastro-intestinal loss. Gastric suction or persistent vomiting results in relatively greater loss of chloride with hydrogen ions than sodium. This leads to hypochloræmic alkalosis. Loss of small intestinal fluid results in relatively greater loss of sodium than chloride.
3. Potassium depletion associated with alkalosis.
4. Sweating with adequate fluid intake, but without added salt.
5. Diabetic ketosis. Although there is chloride loss in the urine associated with the glucose-induced diuresis, there is frequently also severe chloride loss due to vomiting.
6. Renal loss of chloride:—
    a. Renal tubular damage (including sodium loss in salt-losing nephritis).
    b. Mercurial diuretics.
    c. Adrenal cortical deficiency, e.g., Addison's disease.
    d. Cerebral salt wasting after head injury.
    e. Respiratory acidosis.
    f. Excessive sodium bicarbonate intake.
    g. Acute intermittent porphyria.
    h. Variegate porphyria.
7. Paracentesis, e.g., in cirrhosis of the liver with gross ascites.
8. Expansion of the extracellular fluid volume:—
    a. Water intoxication.
    b. Hypothermia, with glucose solution infusion.
    c. Pneumonia.

N.B.—**In bromide intoxication the plasma sodium concentration is unaffected, but the bromide ions replace chloride ions, resulting in hypochloræmia.**

REFERENCES.—Schales, O., and Schales, S. S. (1941), *J. biol. Chem.*, **140**, 879; Wills, M. R., and McGowan, G. K. (1964), *Brit. med. J.*, **1**, 1153.

CHLORIDE IN URINE.—Normally the urine chloride excretion equals the dietary intake.

Average Normal Output.—
    100 mEq./24 hr. (as chloride).
    3·55 g./24 hr. (as chloride).
    5·85 g./24 hr. (as sodium chloride).

Physiological.—
    Increase.—
    1. Increased salt intake.
    2. Post-menstrual diuresis.
    Decrease.—
    1. Reduced salt intake.
    2. Premenstrual salt and water retention.

Pathological.—
    Increase.—
    1. Diuretics, especially chlorothiazide.
    2. Renal tubule damage with gross chloride loss, e.g., salt-losing nephritis, but not usually with other renal damage.

3. Faulty renal tubule salt reabsorption, due to adrenal cortical hormone deficiency (Addison's disease).
4. Potassium depletion.

Decrease.—
1. Low salt diet.
2. Starvation.
3. Excessive chloride loss, due to vomiting, intestinal fistula, or severe diarrhœa.
4. Excessive sweating, with poor sodium chloride intake.
5. Terminal renal disease with oliguria.
6. Both Cushing's syndrome and adrenal steroid therapy result in increased sodium chloride reabsorption by the renal tubules. Post-operative chloride retention is due to the action of excess adrenal steroid hormones.
7. In diabetes insipidus the urine chloride concentration is very low, but because of the large urine volume, the daily output is normal.
8. Any cause of salt retention, e.g., œdema formation, brain damage, etc.

REFERENCE.—Van Slyke, D. D. (1923–4), *J. biol. Chem.*, **58**, 523.

CHOLESTEROL IN SERUM

Normal Range.—
At 1 week.—90–160 mg./100 ml.
At 6 months.—130–210 mg./100 ml.

Adult.—

Age (years)	Males	Females
20	110–250	110–250
30	120–290	120–290
40	135–315	135–290
50	150–340	145–330
60	140–321	156–356
70	140–310	145–380

$$\left(\frac{\text{mg./litre}}{387} = \text{mmol./litre.}\right)$$

The variation is wide between individuals, but the serum cholesterol is relatively constant in any one individual.

The blood cholesterol exists in both a free form and an ester form.

Free Cholesterol.—Equally distributed between plasma and red blood-cells.

Ester Cholesterol.—Occurs only in the plasma. Normally 50–70 per cent of the plasma cholesterol is in the ester form.

Esters
$\begin{cases} 40–50 \text{ per cent as linoleate.} \\ 20–27 \text{ per cent as oleate and palmitoleate.} \\ 12–20 \text{ per cent as palmitate and stearate.} \\ 9–18 \text{ per cent as arachidonate.} \end{cases}$

Although the liver is the main site of esterification, changes occur *in vitro* at room temperature, showing a gradual increase in the ester fraction.

Physiological Variations.—
1. *After Meals.*—Man absorbs cholesterol which is mainly of animal origin, and its absorption from the diet is facilitated

by the presence of neutral fats and bile-salts in the intestines. After absorption in the terminal portion of the ileum, cholesterol takes part in the biosynthesis of steroids and bile salts.

There appear to be a rapid-exchange pool, a slow-exchange pool, and a very slow-exchange pool. During low-cholesterol diets the most active sites of cholesterol synthesis are liver, ileum, and, to a lesser extent, skin. During high-cholesterol feeding, cholesterol synthesis in liver is reduced, but not in other organs.

Interference with the biliary flow increases hepatic cholesterol synthesis, whilst feeding bile-acids reduces cholesterol synthesis but increases cholesterol absorption.

The level of serum cholesterol is not directly related to:—
1. Rate of cholesterol production.
2. Level in rapid-turnover pool (liver plasma, red cells, viscera).
3. Level in slow-turnover pool.

Serum cholesterol is inversely proportional to rate of removal from rapid-turnover pool and metabolic clearance rate of cholesterol.

The rate of production of cholesterol and size of slow-turnover pool are proportional to the body-weight (especially if above normal).

REFERENCE.—Dietschy, J. M., and Wilson, Jean (1970), *New Engl. J. Med.*, **282**, 1241.

2. *In Starvation.*—Variable results are obtained. Cholesterol synthesis is reduced.

3. *Age.*—The pattern of the serum cholesterol level related to age is complicated. After an initial rise after birth, there appears to be a fall in concentration until the middle of the second decade. Thereafter the serum cholesterol level rises steadily with age until the sixth decade, when the level begins to fall. During adult life values in males tend to be higher than in females until after middle age.

4. *Pregnancy.*—In normal pregnancy the serum cholesterol rises to a maximum of about 20–25 per cent above normal by the 30th week. This increase is mainly due to increase in the free cholesterol fraction.

5. *Blood Groups.*—Serum cholesterol tends to be a little higher in Group-A subjects and in $Le^{(a+)}$ than in $Le^{(a-)}$ subjects. There is no difference between Rh positive and Rh negative subjects. It appears that the ester cholesterol fraction is controlled by the blood group.

REFERENCES.—Langman, M. J. S., Elwood, P. C., Foote, J., and Pyrie, D. R. (1969), *Lancet*, **2**, 107; Oliver, M. F., Geizerova, Helena, Cumming, R. A., and Heady, J. A. (1969), *Ibid.*, **2**, 605; Beckman, L., and Olivecrona, T. (1970), *Ibid.*, **1**, 1000.

6. *Experimental Factors.*—
   a. The miscible pool of cholesterol in the body = 0·18–0·35 per cent of body-weight, with a half-life of 58–101 days. Complete equilibration of cholesterol throughout the body, including cholesterol in arterial walls (but not cholesterol in the brain), is attained within 1 month.

  b. High animal fat diets or saturated vegetable fat diets lead to an increase in serum cholesterol.

  c. High unsaturated vegetable diets (e.g., containing sunflower oil, corn oil, or purified linseed oil) or diets containing much untreated fish oils may lead to a fall in serum cholesterol. These oils cause a gross increase in cholic acid excretion in the bile.

7. *Race and Diet.*—In South African Bushmen the serum cholesterol, triglycerides, and phospholipids are normally low.

REFERENCES.—Adlersberg, D., Schaefer, L. E., and Steinberg, A. G. (1956), *J. Amer. med. Ass.*, 162, 619; Lewis, B. (1958), *Lancet*, 1, 1090; Chobanian, A. V., and Hollander, W. (1962), *J. clin. Invest*, 41, 1732; Chobanian, A. V. Burrows, B. A., and Hollander, W. (1962), *Ibid.*, 41, 1738; Taylor, C. B., Mikkelson, B., Anderson, J. A., Forman, D. T., and Choi, S. S. (1965), *Exp. Molec. Path.*, 4/5, 480.

Pathological.—
Increase.—
  1. *Liver Disease.*—
    a. Obstructive Jaundice.—
        i. In simple biliary obstruction the increase is greater in the free fraction.
        ii. Cholangiolitic biliary obstruction.
        iii. Some cases of toxic hepatitis with small biliary duct obstruction.
    b. Hepatic glycogen storage disease (von Gierke's disease).
    c. Mild infective hepatitis and mild portal cirrhosis.
        The variable rise in cholesterol which occurs in these two conditions is mainly in the free fraction.
    d. Primary biliary cirrhosis, greatly increased by clofibrate.

N.B.—Release of obstruction leads to a rapid fall in cholesterol towards normal. The onset of hepatocellular damage during obstruction also leads to a rapid fall in serum cholesterol, but in this latter condition the greater fall is in the ester fraction.

  2. *Renal Disease.*—In the nephrotic stage of nephritis, very high serum cholesterol levels are found.
  3. *Pancreatic Disease.*—
    a. After pancreatectomy.
    b. Some cases of chronic pancreatitis.
    c. Insulin deficiency, i.e., diabetes mellitus.
        If there is associated ketosis, fatty acids are mobilized to form cholesterol. The free/ester ratio remains normal.
  4. *Thyroid Disease.*—The serum cholesterol concentration is increased in hypothyroidism and myxœdema. In true myxœdema the serum cholesterol level is usually more than 200 mg./100 ml., but may be normal if there is also associated malnutrition.
  5. *Xanthomatosis.*
  6. *Idiopathic Hypercholesterolæmia.*—Serum albumin is reduced, whilst the serum gamma globulin fraction is increased. At the same time there is a marked increase in the serum beta-lipoprotein fraction.

Decrease.—

1. *Liver Disease (any case of severe liver damage).—*
    a. Terminal portal cirrhosis.
    b. Acute and subacute hepatic necrosis.
    c. Liver damage due to cinchophen, chloroform, carbon tetrachloride, or phosphorus.
    d. Congestive cardiac failure with severe hepatic congestion.
    e. Infections associated with liver damage, e.g., viral hepatitis, yellow fever, leptospiral infections, and possibly severe pneumonia.

    In severe liver damage the total serum cholesterol falls. In a rapidly fatal case the ester fraction is markedly reduced and may be almost completely absent.

2. *Starvation.*—The level may fall, although this may not occur when there is associated moderate ketosis.

3. *Terminal Uræmia.*—The serum cholesterol may fall, presumably due to the associated poor nutrition.

4. *Severe Sepsis.*—The serum cholesterol may fall. During convalescence the level rises, sometimes above the normal range.

5. *Hyperthyroidism.*—The serum cholesterol concentration falls, but not in simple relation to the associated rise in the basal metabolic rate. Diet has a variable effect on the blood level.

6. *Steatorrhœa.*—Low blood concentrations may be found in some cases.

7. *Cortisone and ACTH Therapy.*—During treatment with either of these substances, the blood level may fall.

8. *Anæmia.—*
    a. Pernicious anæmia. In relapse, the serum cholesterol level is low. During remission, or following treatment, the serum cholesterol increases as the reticulocyte count rises.
    b. Folate deficiency. Serum cholesterol rises following folate treatment.
    c. Hæmolytic anæmia.
    d. Severe hypochromic anæmia.

9. *Hæmophilia.*—The serum total cholesterol may be below normal in this condition.

10. Triparanol inhibits synthesis of cholesterol from its precursor, 24-dehydroxysterol (desmosterol), which increases in the serum.

11. Clofibrate (ethyl-*p*-chlorophenoxyisobutyrate) and androsterone in combination cause reduction of both serum cholesterol and serum triglycerides where the initial serum levels are raised.

12. The lowest serum cholesterol in any disease is found in association with congenital absence of a serum β-lipoprotein.

13. Congenital absence or gross reduction of alpha-lipoprotein, Tangier disease.

14. Severely mentally retarded patients.

15. Familial acyl-transferase deficiency.

16. Œstrogen therapy.
17. Analogues of thyroxine.
18. Nicotinic acid in excessively large doses.
19. Sitosterol in uncomfortably large doses.
20. Resection or by-pass of ileum.

Generally the serum cholesterol is not helpful in diagnosis, but can be used as a rough guide to progress in a given disease process, e.g., myxœdema on thyroid therapy.

REFERENCES.—Sackett, G. E. (1925), *J. biol. Chem.*, **64**, 203; Man, E. B., Kartin, B. L., Durlacher, S. H., and Peters, J. P. (1945), *J. clin. Invest.*, **24**, 623; Oliver, M. F. (1962), *Lancet*, **1**, 1321; Eastham, R. D., and Jancar, J. (1969), *Brit. J. Psychiat.*, **115**, 1013; Bazzano, G. (1970), *Arch. Intern. Med.*, **124**, 710.

FREE AND ESTER CHOLESTEROL IN SERUM

Normal Range.—15–30 per cent of the total serum cholesterol in normal subjects is in the form of non-esterified cholesterol, the remainder being esterified.

Pathological.—Increase in free : ester cholesterol.—

1. Hepatocellular damage, especially in the early phase of infective hepatitis.
2. Familial plasma lecithin : cholesterol acyltransferase deficiency. In this rare condition, the ester cholesterol fraction is virtually absent.

REFERENCES.—Varley, H. (1967), *Practical Clinical Biochemistry*, 4th ed., p. 317. London: Heinemann; Eastham, R. D., Jancar, J., and Lane, R. F. (1971), *Irish J. med. Sci.* In press.

CHOLINESTERASE

CHOLINESTERASE IN RED CELLS ("TRUE CHOLINESTERASE").—

Physiological.—Red-cell concentration two-thirds adult level at birth, reaching normal adult levels by 3 years.

Normal Range.—Cholinesterase number: 51–100 (this represents the fall in pH after 1 hour incubation multiplied by 100). Levels of both red-cell cholinesterase and serum pseudocholinesterase lower in cord blood than normal adult levels.

The red blood-cells contain true cholinesterase which is completely and irreversibly inhibited by organic phosphorus insecticides, e.g., DNOC, parathion, etc. The red-cell cholinesterase level does not rise again to normal after poisoning in under three months, i.e., until newly formed red blood-cells have replaced the damaged ones.

The red blood-cell cholinesterase has been found to be low in untreated pernicious anæmia, increasing to normal following treatment with vitamin B_{12}.

REFERENCE.—Aldridge, W. N., and Davies, D. R. (1952), *Brit. med. J.*, **1**, 945.

CHOLINESTERASE IN SERUM ("PSEUDOCHOLINESTERASE").—

Normal Range.—

1. 0·48 delta pH–1·24 delta pH/hr. incubation (Moore, Birchall, Horack, and Batson, 1957).
2. Cholinesterase number = 40–100 (this represents the pH fall after 1 hour incubation multiplied by 100) (Aldridge and Davies, 1952).

The enzyme appears to be bound to a large mucoprotein molecule associated with the serum albumin and is synthesized by the liver.

Pathological.—

Increase.—

1. During recovery from a relapse in hepatic cirrhosis.
2. During recovery from acute hepatitis.
3. Some cases of thyrotoxicosis. It is not a useful measure of thyroid activity, because of the wide overlap with normal cases.
4. Curare-sensitive patients (i.e., during anæsthesia).
5. Obesity.
6. Diabetes mellitus (obese type).
7. Nephrosis.
8. Alcoholism.
9. Psoriasis (reported).

Decrease.—

1. Liver disease:—
   a. Active cirrhosis.
   b. Acute hepatitis. (May be useful in neonatal jaundice. In hepatitis the level is low, but in pure biliary obstruction the level is normal.)
   c. Carcinomatosis, involving the liver.
2. Cardiac infarction.
3. Malnutrition and chronic debilitating diseases.
4. Severe anæmia, both iron deficiency and pernicious anæmia.
5. Dermatomyositis.
6. Familial idiopathic low plasma cholinesterase. Recently described by Lehmann and others (1958), these cases are excessively sensitive to the action of suxamethonium. They have an unusual form of the enzyme. Homozygotes are extremely sensitive to suxamethonium.
7. Poisoning with organo-phosphorous compounds.
8. Eczema.
9. Phenolzine medication (?).

In general, it appears that the level of this enzyme falls as:—

1. The serum albumin falls.
2. The serum glutamic-oxalacetic transaminase rises.

REFERENCES.—Moore, C. B., Birchall, R., Horack, H. M., and Batson, H. M. (1957), *Amer. J. med. Sci.*, **234**, 538; Lehmann, H., Paston, V., and Ryan, E. (1958), *J. clin. Path.*, **11**, 554; Lehmann, H., and Liddell, J. (1962), *Modern Trends in Anæsthesia* (Ed. Evans and Gray), **2**, p. 164. London: Butterworth; Trotter, M. D., and Fairburn, E. A. (1966), *Brit. J. Dermatol.*, **78**, 469.

COLLOIDAL GOLD REACTIONS

CEREBROSPINAL FLUID COLLOIDAL GOLD REACTION (LANGE CURVE).—Colloidal gold sol is added to a series of dilutions of cerebrospinal fluid. With a normal fluid, only minimal precipitation of the gold sol occurs. Grading the unchanged sol as "0" and the completely precipitated sol as "5", a normal result would read:—

"0 0 0 1 1 0 0 0 0 0".

Gamma-globulin is the principal agent in sol precipitation. Alpha- and beta-globulins inhibit the effect of gamma-globulin, whilst albumin has little inhibitory effect.

Pathological.—

1. *Paretic Type.*—Precipitation occurs in the tubes with the greater concentration of cerebrospinal fluid, i.e., a relatively low albumin concentration in the fluid:—

   "5 5 5 4 3 2 1 0 0 0".

   This type of result is obtained in general paralysis of the insane (G.P.I.) due to syphilis.

2. *Tabetic Type.*—Precipitation occurs in the middle range of tubes, i.e., evidence of partial albumin protection:—

   "1 2 3 3 2 1 0 0 0 0".

   This type of result is obtained in tabes dorsalis due to syphilis.

3. *Meningitic Type.*—Precipitation occurs most in the most dilute tubes, i.e., evidence of greater albumin protection:—

   "0 0 0 1 2 3 3 2 1 0".

   This type of result is obtained in acute meningitis.

4. In disseminated sclerosis when the plaques are near enough to the brain surface to affect the cerebrospinal fluid, paretic curves are obtained.

   In these cases the Wassermann reaction is negative.

5. In treated cases of syphilis of the central nervous system, although the total cerebrospinal protein may be within normal limits, evidence of old disease is found frequently by means of the Lange curve.

6. Encephalomyeloneuropathy due to carcinoma.

   REFERENCES.—Varley, H. (1954), *Practical Clinical Biochemistry.* London: Heinemann; Bloomfield, N. (1964), *Amer. J. clin. Path.,* **41,** 15.

CEREBROSPINAL FLUID COLLOIDAL GOLD REACTION.—

Alternative colloidal suspensions have been used:—

1. *Gum Mastic.*

   REFERENCE.—Cutting, J. A. (1917), *J. Amer. med. Ass.,* **68,** 1810.

2. *Benzoin.*

   REFERENCE.—Evans, N., and Dodson, W. R. (1932), *Amer. J. clin. Path.,* 2, 463.

N.B.—Whatever test is used, the result is not of great practical use. The total cell-count, differential, and total protein in the cerebrospinal fluid are the most useful examinations. Syphilis is detectable by means of the Wassermann reaction applied to the cerebrospinal fluid.

SERUM COLLOIDAL GOLD AND COLLOIDAL RED REACTIONS.—

Normal Result.—0–1, reading as for cerebrospinal fluid Lange curve. The results obtained are roughly parallel with the serum thymol turbidity reaction. The reactions depend on increases in the serum gamma globulin and decreases in the serum albumin concentrations. There appears to be no special advantage over the thymol turbidity reaction. The tests are positive in:—

1. Hepatitis.

2. Hepatic cirrhosis.
3. Carcinomatosis.
4. Severe chronic infections.

REFERENCES.—Maclagan, N. F. (1946), *Brit. J. exp. Path.*, **27**, 190, 369; Maizels, M. (1946), *Lancet*, **2**, 451.

CONGO RED TEST

One hundred mg. of the dye, as 10 ml. of 1 per cent aqueous solution, are injected intravenously into an adult. Normally about 70–90 per cent of the four-minute serum level remains in the serum 60 minutes after the injection. Since there is very rapid removal of congo red from the circulation in amyloid cases during the first few minutes, and since adequate mixing of the dye in the circulation requires at least $7\frac{1}{2}$–20 minutes in normal cases, a much more accurate method has been developed by Unger, Zuckerbrod, Beck, and Steele (1948). The theoretical plasma concentration at zero time is predicted from the estimated plasma volume of the patient and the dose of dye injected. To avoid the complication of lipæmia, the patient should be fasted for 12 hours before the test: 1 ml. of 1 per cent congo red solution/10 lb. body-weight is injected.

Up to 32 per cent of the dye may be removed from the circulation in normal individuals in 30 minutes.

In amyloid disease, more than 35 per cent of the dye is removed in 30 minutes. The persistence in the serum depends on:—

1. There being sufficient albumin present in the serum to bind the dye.
2. Absence of amyloid tissue.
3. Absence of renal leak of the dye.

Reduced Dye Retention in the Serum.—

1. *With no Dye appearing in the Urine.—*Secondary amyloid tissue, occurring in amyloid disease, binds the dye and removes it rapidly from the circulation. Primary amyloid tissue does not bind the dye.
2. *With Dye appearing in the Urine.—*In nephrosis with gross proteinuria, much of the dye is lost bound to the albumin fraction.

N.B.—The injection of congo red solution into patients with a history of asthma or allergy can be extremely dangerous. Evans blue can be safely used to detect amyloid disease. The dye is rapidly taken up by amyloid tissue.

REFERENCES.—Unger, P., Zuckerbrod, M., Beck, G. J., and Steele, J. M. (1948), *J. clin. Invest.*, **27**, 111; Varley, H. (1954), *Practical Clinical Biochemistry*, **131**, 132. London: Heinemann; Jarnum, S., (1960), *Lancet*, **1**, 1007 (describes use of Evans blue).

COPPER

COPPER IN SERUM.—
Normal Range.—68–143 µg./100 ml.
    Males.—$107 \pm 18\cdot2$ µg./100 ml.
    Females.—$118 \pm 25\cdot4$ µg./100 ml.

$$\left(\frac{\mu g./litre}{63\cdot5} = \mu mol./litre.\right)$$

Physiological.—Recently absorbed copper is carried loosely bound to serum albumin, although serum siderophilin may carry a little. After some hours the copper is transferred to the serum alpha-2 globulin cæruloplasmin, the specific copper-carrying protein, which carries 90 per cent of the normal total serum copper.

Since the placenta will not allow the passage of protein-bound maternal copper, the normal maternal/fœtal serum copper ratio is about 8 : 1. The maternal serum copper level rises in the last three months of pregnancy. The serum copper level is low in the normal newborn.

Pathological.—

Increase.—

    1. Acute and chronic infection. It is possible that copper is involved in antibody response.

    2. Acute and chronic leukæmia.

    3. Lymphomas and Hodgkin's lymphadenoma.

    4. Anæmia.—

        a. Aplastic anæmia.

        b. Pernicious anæmia.

        c. Megaloblastic anæmia of pregnancy.

        d. Iron-deficiency anæmia.

    5. Hæmochromatosis.

    6. Hypothyroidism and hyperthyroidism.

    7. Collagen diseases.—

        a. Systemic lupus erythematosus.

        b. Acute rheumatic fever (the serum copper has been used as an index of activity in this disease).

    8. Cirrhosis. Serum copper and cæruloplasmin levels raised.

Raised serum copper levels may indicate either increased cell metabolism or may be a product of cell breakdown.

Decrease.—

    I. Inability to synthesize cæruloplasmin.—

Acute leukæmia in remission induced by either ACTH or prednisone.

    A. Lack of copper.—Iron-deficiency anæmia in some infants. In these infants treatment with iron alone does not cause the hæmoglobin to rise. Copper salts as well as iron salts are necessary for recovery.

    B. Inability to synthesize apoprotein.—

        1. Normal newborn infant.

        2. Hepatolenticular degeneration (Wilson's disease). There is almost complete absence of cæruloplasmin in this condition, and copper is deposited in the liver, brain, and renal tubules.

        3. Kwashiorkor. Associated with low serum iron level.

        4. Sprue in infants.

        5. Cœliac disease in infants.

        6. Idiopathic hypoproteinæmia in infants.

    II. Excessive loss or destruction of cæruloplasmin.—

    A. Excessive loss.—

        1. Nephrosis. Cæruloplasmin is lost in the urine with the massive proteinuria.

        2. Burns.

B. Accelerated rate of protein catabolism.
Transient dysproteinæmia.

REFERENCES.—Lahey, M. E., Gubler, C. J., Chase, M. S., Cartwright, G. E., and Wintrobe, M. M. (1953), *J. clin. Invest.*, **32**, 322, 329; Blomfield, Jeanette, and Macmahan, R. A. (1969), *J. clin. Path.*, **22**, 136.

COPPER OXIDASE ACTIVITY IN SERUM.—

Apart from research into blood formation, etc., the only clinically useful test of copper metabolism is the estimation of serum oxidase activity. Cæruloplasmin will catalyse the oxidation of amines, phenol, and ascorbic acid. The presence of cæruloplasmin in serum excludes a diagnosis of hepatolenticular degeneration.

Physiological.—Serum copper oxidase activity low in newborn. Normal adult levels reached by 6–12 months rising to a peak at 7–9 years, and reaching adult levels again by 10–14 years. (Normal serum cæruloplasmin = 18·5–65·9 mg./100 ml.)

Pathological.—
Increase.—
1. Infection.
2. Carcinoma.
3. Injury. The author found that the serum levels after surgical operation rose unpredictably, and the levels were not related either to plasma fibrinogen increases or to reduction in heparin clotting time.
4. Normal pregnancy.
5. Schizophrenia. Many cases show increased levels.

Decrease.—
1. Hepatolenticular degeneration.
2. Kwashiorkor.
3. Cæruloplasmin reduced in chronic hepatitis.

REFERENCES.—Ravin, H. A. (1961), *J. Lab. clin. Med.*, **58**, 161; Walshe, J. M., and Briggs, J. (1962), *Lancet*, **2**, 263; Sternlieb, I., and Scheinberg, I. H. (1968), *New Engl. J. Med.*, **278**, 352.

COPPER IN URINE.—

Normal Output.—Up to 70 µg./24 hr.
Increased Excretion.—
1. *Defective Serum Protein Binding.*—In hepatolenticular degeneration (Wilson's disease) the cæruloplasmin fraction is defective. Copper is excreted in the urine, bound to amino-acids which act as chelating agents.
2. *Proteinuria.*—Proteinuria results in increased urine copper, since cæruloplasmin appears in the urine in:—
   a. Nephrosis.
   b. Pyelonephritis.
   c. Congestive cardiac failure.
3. *Successful Treatment of Wilson's Disease.*—Gross increase in the urine copper output follows penicillamine therapy. Penicillamine acts as a very effective copper-chelating agent. The urine copper output may be increased by as much as twenty-fold.

N.B.—**The estimation of urine copper is only useful in the assessment of treatment of hepatolenticular degeneration, or diagnosis of this condition.**

COPROPORPHYRIN. *See* **Porphyrins**

CORTICOTROPHIN (ACTH) IN PLASMA

Circulating plasma cortisol damps down the ACTH-releasing factor. This latter substance is thought to be secreted by neural tissue, passing down the hypophysial portal system of vessels to act on the anterior lobe of the pituitary gland, by causing the secretion of corticotrophin. This, in turn, acts on the adrenal cortex, by causing the secretion of cortisol into the circulation.

Physiological.—

Normal values.—There is a normal diurnal rhythm of circulating ACTH in the plasma. The highest values occur between 6 a.m. and 8 a.m. of 22 pg./ml. (0·31 mU./100 ml.), and the lowest values occur between 6 p.m. and midnight, of 10 pg./ml. (0·14 mU./100 ml.). It appears that ACTH has a very short half-life of about 25 minutes.

In normal cord blood the ACTH concentration is greater than the equivalent concentration in the maternal blood at delivery.

Pathological.—

Increased.—

1. Following ACTH injection.
2. Stress.
3. Injury and surgical trauma.
4. Metyrapone injection. After 24–72 hours plasma levels of 70 pg./ml. (1–3 mU./100 ml.) are found.
5. Adrenocortical insufficiency. Plasma levels three to ten times normal are found with low plasma cortisol concentrations.
6. Following adrenalectomy (bilateral).
7. Cushing's syndrome. There is loss of the diurnal rhythm, with the 6 p.m. levels especially being abnormally raised, in spite of abnormally raised plasma cortisol concentrations.
8. Congenital adrenal hyperplasia (0·3–5 mU./100 ml.).
9. Ectopic production by non-pituitary tumours. Levels of 0·5–20 mU./100 ml. may be found in ACTH-secreting carcinomas.
10. Insulin.
11. Lysine-vasopressin.

Decreased.—

1. Steroid suppression. Dexamethasone 0·5 mg. 6-hourly for 2 days is sufficient to suppress circulating ACTH in normal subjects.
2. Panhypopituitarism (less than 0·1 mU./100 ml. plasma).
3. Some adrenocortical tumours.

REFERENCES.—Lipscomb, H. S., and Nelson, D. H. (1962), *Endocrinol.*, **71**, 13; Berson, S. A., and Yalow, R. S. (1968), *J. clin. Invest.*, **47**, 2725; Landon, J., and Greenwood, F. C. (1968), *Lancet*, **1**, 273.

CORTICOTROPHIN STIMULATION TEST

Following intramuscular or intravenous injection of corticotrophin (ACTH) or a synthetic analogue (Synacthen), plasma cortisol concentrations rise and metabolites of cortisol and hydro-cortisol are excreted in the urine as 17-oxogenic steroids.

Twenty-five units of ACTH are given intravenously, or 250 μg. Synacthen are given intramuscularly, after an initial heparinized plasma sample has been taken from the patient. Further heparinized blood samples are taken at 30 minutes and 60 minutes.

Normal Results.—
Fasting plasma cortisol 7·2–25·8 μg./100 ml.
30-minute plasma cortisol 7·7–26·1 μg./100 ml.
60-minute plasma cortisol 21·5–44·0 μg./100 ml.

Pathological.—Fasting plasma cortisol grossly increased, *see* possible causes under 11-Hydroxycorticosteroids in Plasma.

Subsequent samples.—Plasma cortisol concentration fails to rise by more than +2·6 μg./100 ml. in—
   a. Adrenocortical failure.
   b. Hypopituitarism with secondary adrenal depression.

REFERENCE.—Greig, W. R., Boyle, J. A., Maxwell, J. D., Lindsay, R. M., and Browning, Margaret (1969), *Postgrad. med. J.*, **45**, 307.

Intramuscular Test followed by urine estimations.—Thirty units of ACTH are injected intramuscularly three times daily for 3 days, and 24-hr. urine samples are collected each day.

Normal.—The urine excretion of 17-oxogenic steroids increases by 20–60 mg./24 hr. above the initial base-line 24-hr. excretion rate.

Abnormal.—The urine excretion of 17-oxogenic steroids increases by less than 3 mg./24 hr. or remains unchanged.—
   a. Adrenocortical failure.
   b. Hypopituitarism with secondary adrenal depression.

(If facilities for plasma cortisol estimations are available, the first test is preferred, since results are obtained more quickly, and the necessity for 24-hr. urine collections with their associated errors is avoided.)

CORTISOL IN PLASMA. *See* 17-Hydroxycorticosteroids

CREATINE

CREATINE TOLERANCE TEST.—A test dose of 1·32 g. of creatine hydrate is given orally. Normally, creatine is taken up by the muscle cells until they are saturated.

Normal Results.—
   1. *Adult Male.*—80 per cent is retained. Less than 20 per cent appears in the 24-hr. urine specimen.
   2. *Adult Female.*—70 per cent is retained. Less than 30 per cent appears in the 24-hr. urine specimen.

Reduced Tolerance (Increased urine creatine excretion).—When the muscle mass is reduced, or is unable to take up creatine.—
   1. Hyperthyroidism.
   2. Muscle wasting.—
      a. Primary muscle dystrophies.
      b. Secondary muscle dystrophies.

3. Hypothyroidism treated successfully with thyroid extract.
Increased Tolerance (Reduced urine creatine excretion).—
Hypothyroidism. This test may be useful in the detection of cretinism.

N.B.—The creatine tolerance may be normal in myotonia, and in some cases of myasthenia gravis.

REFERENCE.—Richardson, H. B., and Shorr, E. (1935), *Trans. Ass. Amer. Physns*, **50**, 156.

CREATINE IN SERUM.—
Normal Range.—0·2–0·6 mg./100 ml.

$$\left(\frac{mg./litre}{131} = mmol./litre.\right)$$

Since red blood-cells contain about ten times this amount, it is essential to avoid hæmolysis when the blood specimen is collected.

Increase.—
1. Increased ingestion in diet (high meat diet).
2. Increased liver synthesis of creatine (methyl testosterone therapy).
3. Muscle mass destruction.
4. Reduced muscle mass (e.g., limb amputation).
5. Hyperthyroidism.
6. Rheumatoid arthritis, in an active phase.
7. Intravenous injection of enzymatic hydrolysate of casein.

Decrease.—The amounts normally present in serum are too small for a lower limit of normal to be recognized.

REFERENCE.—Brod, J., and Sirota, J. H. (1948), *J. clin. Invest.*, **27**, 645.

CREATINE IN URINE.—
Normal Urine Output.—
1. At 1 month—9 mg./kg. body-weight.
2. At 6 years—4 mg./kg. body-weight.
3. At 10 years—2 mg./kg. body-weight.
4. Boys produce a normal adult urine creatine/creatinine ratio at about 7 years of age. Girls continue to excrete more than boys until puberty, and then show levels of excretion fluctuating with menstruation, until the menopause.
5. Average adult.—Total output of 0–50 mg./24 hr.

Creatine is normally present only in traces in adult urine. The kidney tubules reabsorb filtered creatine.

Physiological.—
Increase.—
1. Normal growing children.
2. Pregnancy. It has been suggested that renal tubule reabsorption is depressed.
3. Early puerperium (2 weeks). Probably the excess creatine is derived from involuting uterine muscle.
4. Severe protein fast, i.e., there is some body muscle protein breakdown.
5. High raw meat diet (cooking converts much of the creatine in the muscle cells to creatinine).
6. Intravenous injection of enzymatic hydrolysate of casein.

Pathological.—

Increase.—

1. *Increased Formation.—*
    a. Myopathies.—
        i. Primary, e.g., amyotonia congenita.
        ii. Secondary, e.g., poliomyelitis.
        iii. Myoglobinuria:—
            α. Muscle destruction after crush injury.
            β. Muscle breakdown in acute paroxysmal myo-globinuria.
    b. Endocrine disorders.—
        i. Hyperthyroidism and excess thyroxine therapy.
        ii. Addison's disease.
        iii. Eunuchoidism and castrates.
        iv. ACTH and cortisone therapy.
        v. Methyl testosterone therapy. Both the production and storage of creatine is encouraged.
    c. Other causes.—
        i. Infections (increased body protein catabolism).
        ii. Secondary carcinoma of the liver.
        iii. Disseminated lupus erythematosus.
        iv. Burns.
        v. Bone fractures.
        vi. Acute leukæmia and active subacute myeloid leukæmia.
2. *Increased Formation and Decreased Renal Reabsorption.—*
    a. Diabetes mellitus.
    b. Acromegaly.
    c. Cushing's syndrome.
    d. Post-DOCA therapy.

Decrease.—

1. Cretin (hypothyroid). The urine contains little or no creatine.
2. Testosterone therapy. The storage of creatine in muscle is stimulated; cf. effect of methyl testosterone.

N.B.—In dermatomyositis and scleroderma the hippuric acid excretion test is normal, if renal function is normal. Therefore the body has plenty of available glycine.

In myotonic dystrophy both the urine creatine and creatinine are less than expected for the muscle mass. This suggests that the rate of creatine synthesis is depressed.

REFERENCE.—Bosnes, R. W., and Taussky, H. H. (1945), *J. biol. Chem.* **158**, 581.

CREATINE PHOSPHOKINASE IN CEREBROSPINAL FLUID

Normal Results.—In the newborn infant results less than 2·5 i.u./litre are found.

Pathological.—

*Increase.—*In newborn infants with levels greater than 2–5 i.u./litre there has been found actual or eventual evidence of brain damage.

REFERENCE.—Belton, N. R. (1970), *Amer. J. clin. Path.*, **45**, 600.

CREATINE PHOSPHOKINASE IN SERUM

The enzyme catalyses the reaction:—
$$Creatine + ATP \rightleftharpoons Creatine\ phosphate + ADP.$$
The highest tissue concentrations of the enzyme are found in heart muscle, skeletal muscle, and brain tissue.

Normal Range.—0·3–4·5 μmoles creatine/ml./hr. at 37° C.; 10–60 i.u./litre (check range with method used). Although moderate exercise has no effect, severe physical exertion causes a marked rise in serum levels persisting for 1–2 days. Raised at birth, the adult level is reached after the first month.

Serum levels are increased at 8–16 hours after exercise, in the absence of training. After proper training, there is little or no increase. There is rapid loss of creatine phosphokinase activity in serum stored at 4° C., probably due to copper oxidase activity. Activity is restored by addition of cysteine, glutathione, etc. Methods using such activation give more clinically significant results in muscular dystrophy and myocardial infarction. Results obtained depend very much on the method of estimation.

REFERENCES.—Vejjajiva, A., and Teasdale, G. M. (1965), *Brit. med. J.*, **1**, 1653; Nuttall, F. Q., and Jones, B. (1968), *J. Lab. clin. Med.*, **71**, 847; Kierkegaard-Hansen, A., and Kierkegaard-Hansen, G. (1969), *Dan. med. Bull.*, **16**, 53; Crowley, L. V., and Alton, Mary (1970), *Amer. J. clin. Path.*, **53**, 948.

Pathological.—
Increase.—
1. *Myocardial Infarction.*—The serum level increases by 3 hours, reaching peak values by 36 hours (10–25 times upper limit of normal), returning to normal values by 4 days. Prolonged elevation is an indication of a bad prognosis.
2. *Progressive Muscular Dystrophy.*—Range of values up to 50 times normal upper limit with higher results in the younger patients. Some mothers of cases of progressive muscular atrophy have increased serum levels, especially in the severe form of the disease, but all fathers so far examined have normal levels. Abnormal results are accentuated if vasoconstriction is applied for 10 minutes before venesection.

   (Muscular atrophy of neurogenic origin shows no such increase in serum levels.)
3. *Muscle Crush Injury.*—The serum level is raised for about 15 days, especially if there is associated arterial obstruction.
4. Cerebral vascular accident. Peak values occur at 48 hours, falling in 3–4 days. Bad prognosis is indicated by an early rise, and by its magnitude. No increase is associated with brain-stem infarction or angiomata.
5. Necrotic glioma.
6. Cerebral ischæmia, and cerebral anoxia, especially after status epilepticus.
7. Hypothermia, from damage to skeletal and cardiac muscle.
8. Tetanus.
9. Carbon-monoxide poisoning.

10. Treatment of amœbic dysentery with emetine.
11. Clofibrate therapy (early stages).
12. Following direct-current countershock to convert arrhythmia, as a result of damage to intercostal muscles.
13. Carbenoxolone therapy (rarely).
14. Hypothyroidism. Abnormally high serum levels are found. (The enzyme is inhibited by thyroxine.)
15. Chronic alcoholism.
16. Malignant hyperpyrexia following anæsthesia. The tendency to develop this condition is inherited as an autosomal dominant character.

REFERENCE.—Denborough, M. A., Forster, J. F. A., Hudson, M. C., and Carter, N. G. (1970), *Lancet*, **1**, 1137.

17. Following intramuscular injection of ampicillin or carbenicillin, due to skeletal muscle damage.

REFERENCES.—Hughes, B. P. (1962), *Clin. chim. Acta*, **7**, 597; Hughes, B. P. (1962), *Brit. med. J.*, **2**, 963; Wilson, K. M., Evans, K. A., and Carter, C. (1965), *Ibid.*, **1**, 750; Nygren, A. (1966), *Acta med. scand.*, **179**, 623; Eisen, A. A., and Sherwin, A. L. (1968), *Neurology*, **18**, 263; Hunt, D., and Bailie, M. J. (1968), *Amer. Heart J.*, **76**, 340; Maclean, D., Griffiths, P. D., and Emslie-Smith, D. (1968), *Lancet*, **2**, 1266.

Red blood-cells do not contain this enzyme, and there is no increase in serum levels in liver disease or biliary obstruction. It would therefore seem to be a useful test in early suspected myocardial infarction, as well as in early progressive muscular atrophy.

CREATININE

PLASMA CREATININE CLEARANCE.—

1. Endogenous Creatinine Clearance.—In addition to glomerular filtration, renal tubular excretion of creatinine also occurs. The usual chemical estimation of blood creatinine includes other chromogens. Hence the fortuitous result is that the endogenous creatinine clearance (if the blood creatinine level is normal) may approximate to the true glomerular filtration rate.

The endogenous clearance is only useful as a rough guide to the glomerular filtration rate *if* renal function is normal. This is because it has been found that in renal failure, the endogenous creatinine clearance is higher than the simultaneously estimated inulin clearance, i.e., there is increased tubular creatinine secretion as the glomerular filtered fraction is reduced. There is a large discrepancy only when the glomerular filtration rate is low (i.e., when the variation is less important).

In hypertensives the daily production of creatinine, and hence clearance, is greater than in normotensives with the same degree of renal damage. With declining glomerular filtration, the creatinine clearance overestimates glomerular function (i.e., increasing tubular secretion of creatinine).

The endogenous creatinine clearance is decreased in old age, even though the plasma creatinine may be within normal limits.

2. Exogenous Creatinine Clearance.—From 3 to 5 g. of creatinine in 400 ml. water are given orally. Two samples of blood are collected during the period of urine collection. Since there is a relative excess of creatinine, the effect of non-specific chromogens on the serum creatinine estimation is reduced. Also, as the serum creatinine level rises, so tubular secretion of creatinine increases. The result is that high creatinine clearance values are obtained. The normal range of 100–200 ml. per minute is very large, and for this reason this test cannot be regarded as a sensitive one.

N.B.—**Treatment with ACTH, cortisone, or thyroxine should be stopped before either test is made.**

3. Plasma Phosphate/Plasma Creatinine Clearance Ratio.—

Increase.—

1. Primary hyperparathyroidism.
2. Osteomalacia.
3. Uræmia (frequently).
4. Idiopathic hypercalcuria.
5. Malignant disease with hypercalcæmia.
6. Cushing's syndrome.

Decrease.—

Hypoparathyroidism.

REFERENCES.—Camara, A. A., Arn, K. D., Reimer, A., and Newburgh, L. H. (1951), *J. Lab. clin. Med.*, **37**, 743; Hansen, J. M., Kampmann, J., and Laursen, H. (1968), *Lancet*, **1**, 1170; Hilden, M., and Hilden, T. (1968), *Acta med. scand.*, **183**, 183; Kim, K. E., Onesti, G., Ramirez, O., Brest, A. N., and Swartz, C. (1969), *Brit. med. J.*, **4**, 11.

CREATININE IN SERUM.—

Normal Range.—0·9–1·7 mg./100 ml. (proportional to body size).

$$\left(\frac{\text{mg./litre}}{113} = \text{mmol./litre.} \right)$$

Creatinine is formed from creatine, and diffuses freely throughout the body water. Unlike creatine, it is a waste product.

On a creatinine-free diet, the daily production and excretion of creatinine is constant, is proportional to the body muscle mass, and corresponds approximately to 2 per cent of the total body creatine.

Physiological.—

Increase.—After ingestion of creatinine (e.g., roast meats).

Pathological.—

Increase.—

1. Increased rate of formation.—
   a. Gigantism.
   b. Acromegaly.
2. Diminished renal excretion of creatinine.—
   a. Renal failure.
   b. Uræmia.
   c. Severe congestive cardiac failure.

N.B.—**The serum creatinine level often increases after the blood-urea has increased, when extensive damage to the kidneys has occurred.**

REFERENCE.—Brod, J., and Sirota, J. H. (1948), *J. clin. Invest.*, **27**, 645.

CREATININE IN URINE.—

On a creatinine-free diet the daily urine excretion is constant, and directly related to the total body mass of muscle. The 24-hr. output is not sufficiently constant to justify its use as a reference for the excretion rates of other substances.

Normal Output.—
  Adult male—1·5–2·0 g./24 hours ⎱ Proportional to
  Adult female—0·8–1·5 g./24 hours ⎰ body-size
Approximately 15–25 mg./kg. body-weight/24 hr.

Normal Output for Children.—
  1 week—5 mg./kg. body-weight/24 hr.
  6 months—12 mg./kg. body-weight/24 hr.
  6 years—15 mg./kg. body-weight/24 hr.

Physiological.—
  Increase.—The urine creatinine increases after ingestion of creatinine-rich foods, e.g., roast meats, especially the outer slices.

Pathological.—
  Increase.—
    1. Acromegaly.
    2. Gigantism.
    3. Diabetes mellitus.
    4. Infections.
    5. Hypothyroidism (with associated fall in urine creatine).
  Decrease.—
    1. Hyperthyroidism (with associated rise in urine creatine).
    2. Anæmia.
    3. Paralysis.
    4. Muscle atrophy.
    5. Active dermatomyositis. As the urine creatine increases, so the urine creatinine falls.
    6. Advanced renal disease, before the final stage of failure.
    7. Leukæmia, returning towards normal in remission.

REFERENCES.—Bosnes, H. W., and Taussky, H. H. (1945), *J. biol. Chem.*, **158**, 581; Paterson, N. (1967), *Clin. chim. Acta*, **18**, 57; Edwards, O. M., Bayliss, R. I. S., and Millen, S. (1969), *Lancet*, **2**, 1165.

DEXAMETHASONE SUPPRESSION TEST

1. URINE TESTS.—Two control 24-hr. urine samples are collected. Then 2 mg. dexamethasone are given orally every 6 hours for a total of eight doses. Two further 24-hr. urine samples are collected during the test.

Normal.—Urine total 17-oxogenic steroid output falls to less than 2·5 mg./24 hr.

Pathological.—In Cushing's syndrome due either to adrenal hyperplasia or to adrenal adenoma, the response ranges from no fall in output to a marked fall in urine output of total 17-oxogenic steroids. When Cushing's syndrome is due to adrenal carcinoma, there is usually no fall in the abnormally raised urine output of total 17-oxogenic steroids.

2. PLASMA CORTISOL TESTS.—Control plasma 11-hydroxy-corticosteroid samples are taken at 9 a.m. and at 11 p.m. At midnight 1 mg. of dexamethasone is given in saline intravenously over a 3-hour period.

Normal.—At 8–9 a.m. the plasma 11-hydroxycorticosteroid level has fallen below 6 μg./100 ml.

Abnormal (no fall in plasma levels).—
    1. Severe illness.
    2. Oestrogens and oral contraceptives.

3. Encephalitis.

4. Complicated diabetes mellitus.

5. Cushing's syndrome. Plasma levels may exceed 20 $\mu g./$ 100 ml. If a 2-mg. dose is given, this may or may not cause a fall in plasma levels in benign hyperplasia. If the dose is increased to 4 or 8 mg., plasma levels usually (but not always) fall in benign hyperplasia. When Cushing's syndrome is due to an adrenal tumour, plasma levels usually do not fall.

Alternatively.—

Normal.—Plasma 11-hydroxycorticosteroids fall to 23–37 per cent of resting level 3 hours after 1 mg. intravenous dexamethasone.

Pathological.—

Adrenal hyperplasia.—Fall in plasma levels no further than to 44 per cent of resting level.

Adrenal tumour.—No fall in plasma levels after 3 hours.

DUODENAL INTUBATION
(Associated with Pancreatic Stimulation)

After passage of a duodenal tube, secretin (1 unit/kg. body-weight) is injected intravenously. Subsequently two samples at 10-minute intervals and two further samples at 20-minute intervals are aspirated. Secretin stimulation merely "washes out" the ducts in the gland.

At the end of the first hour, pancreozymin (1·5 units/kg. body-weight) is injected slowly intravenously. Two samples of duodenal juice are then aspirated at 10-minute intervals.

Normal.—

1. *Normal Volume.*—206 ± 54 ml. in 80-minute period.

2. *Bicarbonate Excretion.*—13·5 ± 4·6 mEq. in 80-minute period.

3. *Amylase Excretion.*—559 ± 280 units in 80-minute period.

REFERENCE.—Lagerlof, H. O. (1942), *Acta med. scand.*, Suppl., **128**, 1.

4. *Trypsin Excretion.*—14,020 ± 8300 units in 80-minute period.

REFERENCE.—Gowenlock, A. H. (1953), *Biochem. J.*, **53**, 274.

5. *Lipase Excretion.*—6260 ± 1580 units in 80-minute period.

REFERENCE.—Sammons, H. G., Frazer, A. C., and Thompson, M. (1956), *J. clin. Path.*, **9**, 379.

Pathological.—Reduced secretion of pancreatic juice and reduced enzyme concentration results from:—

1. Obstruction to the pancreatic duct:—
   a. Calculus.
   b. Carcinoma of pancreas.
   c. Fibrosis, as in recurrent pancreatitis.
   d. Fibrocystic disease of the pancreas.

2. Diminished power to secrete enzymes:—
   a. Pancreatitis.
   b. Congenital deficiency of pancreatic lipase.

N.B.—**The technique of duodenal intubation is not easy, and the test is time-consuming.**

REFERENCES.—Howat. H. T. (1952), *Pancreatitis, Modern Trends in Gastroenterology* (Ed. Avery-Jones, F.). London : Butterworth; Marks, I. N., and Tompsett, S. L. (1958), *Quart. J. Med.*, **27**, 431.

FAT

FAT IN CEREBROSPINAL FLUID.—No significant difference has been found in fat globules in the cerebrospinal fluid in traumatic and non-traumatic cases with neurological signs or symptoms.

REFERENCE.—Tedeschi, C. G., Walter, C. E., Lepore, T., and Tedeschi, L. G. (1969), *Neurology (Minn.)*, **19**, 586.

FAT IN FÆCES.—

Normal Output.—

1. *Analysis of a Single Specimen.—*

   Infant.—Less than 50 per cent of fæcal dry weight. (⅔ split.)

   Adult.—Less than 25 per cent of fæcal dry weight. (¾ split.)

2. *Analysis of 24-hour Specimens.*—A general average diet contains 50–100 g. of fat per diem. In the normal, 90–95 per cent of this fat is absorbed. The fat excreted in the stool (expressed as fatty acid) should not exceed more than 5 g./24 hr. averaged over three consecutive 24-hr. periods.

   An excretion of more than 4 g. per diem is abnormal in a child.

N.B.—Wherever possible, analysis of 24-hr. specimens is preferable to the analysis of isolated specimens. The total amount of fat excreted is far more important than the amount of split/unsplit fat in the specimen.

Pathological.—

Increase: *Steatorrhœa.—*

1. Excessively rapid passage of intestinal contents:—
   a. Severe diarrhœa.
   b. Gastrocolic fistula.
2. Biliary disease:—
   a. Obstruction of the common bile-duct.
   b. External bile fistula.
   c. Congenital absence of bile-salts.
   d. Congenital absence of pancreatic lipase.
3. Pancreatic disease:—
   a. Chronic pancreatitis (often high fæcal nitrogen output if severe).
   b. Obstruction to the pancreatic duct (the enzyme lipase is unable to reach the intestine).
4. Obstruction to lymphatic flow from the intestines:—
   a. Lymphoma, e.g., lymphosarcoma, Hodgkin's disease.
5. Impaired absorption:—
   a. Allergy to gluten (wheat protein), as in cœliac disease.
   b. Non-tropical idiopathic steatorrhœa.
   c. Tropical sprue.
   d. Whipple's disease.
   e. Postgastrectomy (more severe after Polya than Billroth operation).
   f. Hypoadrenocorticalism (Addison's disease). Replacement steroid therapy results in disappearance of steatorrhœa.
   g. Neomycin. Transient steatorrhœa may follow large doses of neomycin.
   h. Zollinger-Ellison syndrome. Steatorrhœa may occur.
   i. Carcinoid syndrome controlled by means of serotonin antagonists may develop steatorrhœa.

j. Total and anterior selective vagotomy.

k. Pyloroplasty (with reduced stool colour and increased bowel frequency).

REFERENCES.—Weyers, H. A., and Van de Kamer, J. H. (1949), *J. biol. Chem.*, **177**, 347; Frazer, A. C. (1955), *Brit. med. J.*, **2**, 805; Badenoch, J. (1960), *Ibid.*, **2**, 879 and 963 (review of adult steatorrhœa with 157 references); McBrien, D. J., Jones, R. V., and Creamer, B. (1963), *Lancet*, **1**, 25; Sheldon, W. (1964), *Arch. Dis. Childh.*, **39**, 268; Wastell, C., and Ellis, H. (1966), *Brit. med. J.*, **1**, 1195.

FIBRINOGEN IN PLASMA

Normal Range.—200–400 mg./100 ml. It is probable that fibrinogen is formed entirely in the liver. Hepatectomy in the experimental animal leads to a progressive fall in the plasma fibrinogen. Pus from sterile abscesses in experimental animals contains a factor which stimulates fibrinogen formation.

Plasma fibrinogen tends to be low in normal newborn infant. A normal moderate increase occurs both during pregnancy and at menstruation.

The plasma level remains fairly constant in an individual in the absence of illness, etc., but fibrinogen turnover increases with age and with increasing vascular degeneration.

Pathological.—

Increase.—
1. Acute infection.
2. Trauma. Maximum increase between fifth and tenth days after surgical operation.
3. After myocardial infarction.
4. Collagen diseases. The plasma fibrinogen has been used to assess activity in both rheumatic carditis and rheumatoid arthritis.
5. Nephrosis. A very high concentration may be found.
6. Hepatitis (in the absence of severe liver damage).
7. Post X-ray therapy (indicates tissue damage).
8. Burns (response to tissue injury).
9. Myeloma (some cases).
10. Scurvy.

Decrease.—
1. *Depressed Formation.*—
   a. Liver failure, especially in severe biliary cirrhosis.
   b. Severe cachectic states.
   c. Moderate depression occurs in:—
      i. Pernicious anæmia.
      ii. Pellagra.
      iii. Scurvy.
      iv. Myeloid leukæmia.
      v. Bone-marrow disorders.
      vi. Polycythæmia vera.
      vii. Typhoid fever (it has been reported in this condition).
      viii. Severe heat-stroke.
2. *Excessive Utilization.*—Due to release of tissue thromboplastin:—
   a. Ante-, intra-, and post-partum hæmorrhage.

    b. Amniotic fluid embolism.
    c. Retention of dead fœtus in utero.
    d. In association with hydatidiform mole.
    e. After incompatible blood transfusion.
    f. Perfusion by extracorporeal pump.
    g. Pulmonary manipulation at operation.
    h. Severe shock, during operation, or after trauma.
    i. Anticoagulant treatment with venom of Malayan pit-viper (Arvin).

3. *Congenital Absence of Fibrinogen.*—The congenital absence of fibrinogen is due to the action of a rare recessive gene.

4. *Dysfibrinogenœmia.*—Rare congenital functional abnormality.

REFERENCE.—King, E. J., and Wootton, I. D. P. (1956), *Micro-analysis in Medical Biochemistry*, 3rd ed., 50–54. London : J. & A. Churchill.

GALACTOSE TOLERANCE TESTS

Galactose is metabolized mainly in the liver. Its renal threshold is low.

N.B.—**The blood galactose is raised in cases of galactosæmia, but the performance of the tolerance test in these cases is dangerous and should not be done, as severe hypoglycæmia accompanies the rise in blood galactose.**

ORAL TOLERANCE TEST.

1. Forty g. galactose in water are given orally after an overnight fast.
2. Urine samples are collected hourly for 5 hours.
3. Blood is collected fasting and ½-hourly for 2 hours.

Results.—

1. *Urine Output.*—Normally up to 3 g. of galactose are excreted in the urine. A urine output of more than 3 g. of galactose suggests hepatocellular damage.
2. *Blood Levels.—*
    a. The sum of the four blood galactose concentrations normally falls within a total of 0–110 mg.
      i. In acute hepatitis the figure may exceed 500 mg.
      ii. Cirrhosis of the liver. The result may be 400–500 mg.
    b. The normal rise in the blood galactose reaches a peak of 15–35 mg./100 ml., and falls to zero within 2 hours.
      i. Hyperthyroidism. The blood galactose peak reaches 25–150 mg./100 ml.
      ii. In the absence of hyperthyroidism, a blood galactose level of more than 40 mg./100 ml. suggests liver damage.
      iii. Diminished tolerance may also occur in hyperpituitarism.

GASTRIC TEST MEAL

WITH TUBE.—No food should be taken from the previous evening onwards, until the test has been completed next morning. The gruel test-meal has been superseded by the augmented histamine test.

1. **Fasting Specimen.—**
   a. *Volume.*—The specimen is abnormal if the volume is greater than 100–200 ml. The presence of lactic acid indicates stasis, low hydrochloric acid content, and fermentation. There may be evidence of previous meals, e.g., tomato skins. There should be no trace of two charcoal biscuits eaten on the previous night. Gastric emptying is slower if a gastric ulcer is present.
   b. *Blood.*—A little fresh blood may be present in the fasting specimen due to passage of the tube. Otherwise a larger quantity, which may be reddish-brown, suggests gastric bleeding, if bleeding from the nose, mouth, or gums can be excluded. Gastric bleeding occurs in:—
      i. Simple gastritis.
      ii. Benign gastric ulcer.
      iii. Gastric carcinoma.
   c. *Mucus.*—The presence of much mucus, if the swallowing of saliva can be excluded, suggests gastritis or carcinoma.

2. **Overnight Aspiration** (6 p.m.–6 a.m.).—
   Volume.—140–1200 ml. (very wide normal range). Hydrochloric acid: 10–3500 mg. (very wide normal range).

3. **Basal Gastric Secretion.—**
   Males—$1\cdot3\pm1\cdot6$ mEq./hr.
   Females—$1\cdot1\pm1\cdot75$ mEq./hr.

4. **Augmented Histamine Test-meal.—**By giving antihistamines to protect the patient from unpleasant side-effects, it is possible to give larger doses of histamine (0·04 mg. per kg. body-weight). There is a direct relationship between the maximum acid output and the total number of parietal cells in the stomach. This is a much more stringent test of absolute achlorhydria. Normal maximum output of hydrochloric acid in males is $10\cdot8\pm6\cdot9$ mEq. in $\frac{1}{2}$ hr.; in females $6\cdot1\pm4\cdot4$ mEq. in $\frac{1}{2}$ hr. In duodenal ulcer this rate is increased to 22·9 mEq. in $\frac{1}{2}$ hr., whilst in gastric ulcer the maximum rate is 13·1 mEq. in $\frac{1}{2}$ hr. Stimulated acid output of more than 20 mEq./hr. is suggestive evidence against gastric carcinoma. In the Zollinger-Ellison syndrome the unstimulated rate is >40 per cent of the maximum stimulated rate of acid output. A similar high ratio is found when there are antral remnants after partial gastrectomy. After vagotomy pepsin output is reduced, but total chloride secretion is unchanged.

   Achlorhydria occurs in:—
   a. Gastritis.
   b. Gastric carcinoma (some cases).
   c. Severe debility, e.g., advanced tuberculosis, Addison's disease.
   d. Women suffering from iron-deficiency anæmia.
   e. Patients with pernicious anæmia, and many of their relatives.
   f. Many normal old people.
   g. Hypothyroidism. 40–50 per cent of patients have achlorhydria plus intrinsic factor failure.

REFERENCE.—Kay, A. W. (1953), *Brit. med. J.*, **2**, 77.

5. Intrinsic Factor.—Presence or absence of intrinsic factor can be demonstrated by estimation of the rate of absorption of radioactive tagged vitamin B_{12}.

REFERENCE.—Chanarin, I. (1968), *Gut*, **9**, 373.

6. Pentagastrin Test.—This pentapeptide may be used in place of histamine to induce acid secretion.

REFERENCE.—Mason, M. C., and Giles, G. R. (1969), *Gut*, **10**, 375.

TUBELESS TEST-MEALS.—These tests depend on the liberation of quinine from either a quinine salt or a quinine-resin complex by free gastric hydrochloric acid. They may be useful in screening surveys, but for accurate clinical assessment the augmented histamine test-meal, which measures the maximal gastric secretion rate directly, is to be preferred.

GASTRIN IN SERUM

Normal Range.—5–290 pg./ml. (measured by radio-immuno-assay).
Physiological.—
 Increase.—After food.
 Decrease.—After secretin.
Pathological.—
 Decrease.—Post-vagotomy.
 Increase.—
  1. Pernicious anæmia, e.g., 5000 pg./ml.
  2. Zollinger-Ellison syndrome, e.g., 2800–5000 pg./ml.
  3. Duodenal ulcer.

REFERENCES.—Byrnes, D. J., Young, J. D., Chisholm, D. J., and Lazarus, L. (1970), *Brit. med. J.*, **2**, 626; Hansky, J., and Cain, M. D. (1970), *Lancet*, **2**, 1388.

GLOMERULAR FILTRATION RATE (GFR)

Inulin is freely filtered by the renal glomeruli. The concentrations in the plasma and the filtrate are equal. Since the tubules neither reabsorb nor actively secrete inulin, the glomerular filtration rate can be measured:—

$$\frac{\text{Minute excretion of inulin in urine (mg.)}}{\text{Plasma inulin concentration (mg./ml.)}} = \text{GFR}.$$

The normal glomerular filtration rate = 130 ml./min. per 1·73 sq. m. body-surface. This applies only over the age of 2 years, and the GFR is much lower at birth. The GFR of infants is much nearer the adult level if expressed per unit of body water or body-weight; it reaches adult levels in a few weeks, and is above adult levels at the age of 2 years.

Both inulin and creatinine can be used to estimate the glomerular filtration rate, higher readings being obtained with creatinine than inulin in the presence of impaired renal function. It appears that very accurate measurements can be obtained using radioactive vitamin B_{12} (tagged with ^{58}Co).

N.B.—**The GFR per unit of total body water reaches adult levels by the second week after birth.**
Physiological.—
 Decrease.—
  1. The GFR falls proportionally to the severity of muscular exercise.

2. The GFR falls if the dietary protein is reduced.
3. The GFR is lower at night than during the day.
4. The GFR decreases in old age.

Increase.—
1. High protein diet.
2. Intravenous hypertonic saline (10 per cent) may raise the normal GFR to 285 ml./min.

Pathological.—

Decrease.—
1. Renal blood-flow reduced:—
   a. After shock.
   b. After hæmorrhage.
   c. Severe dehydration.
   d. In severe congestive cardiac failure.
2. Reduced effective filtration pressure:—
   a. Decrease in afferent glomerular blood-pressure.
   b. Increase in efferent glomerular blood-pressure.
3. Reduced filtration surface: i.e., reduced number of functioning glomeruli:—
   a. Glomerulonephritis.
   b. Nephrosclerosis.
   c. Pyelonephritis.
   d. Amyloidosis, etc.
4. Hepatorenal failure.—In severe obstructive jaundice the GFR is reduced. There is an increased tendency to develop renal failure following surgery.
5. The plasma protein colloid pressure may vary sufficiently to affect the GFR. This is unlikely, since the plasma protein changes in disease are most frequently a fall in albumin and a rise in the globulin fraction. This might theoretically tend to increase the GFR, e.g., in nephrosis.

It is not known for certain whether sodium thiosulphate can be used for the accurate measurement of the GFR in man. (This substance is actively secreted by the tubule cells of the kidneys in dogs.)

The following substances are probably secreted by the kidney in man in the same manner as inulin:—
   a. Sucrose (do not use, as it can cause renal damage).
   b. Raffinose.
   c. Sorbitol.
   d. Mannite (about 10 per cent of the mannite filtered by the glomeruli is probably reabsorbed by the tubules).
   e. Dulcite.

In practice, thiosulphate and inulin are the substances usually used.

Recently it has been found that the average of the urea and creatinine clearance agrees with the inulin clearance throughout the whole range of the GFR.

REFERENCES.—Dawson, J. L. (1968), *Ann. R. Coll. Surg.*, **42**, 163; Lavender, S., Hilton, P. J., and Jones, N. F. (1969), *Lancet*, **2**. 1216.

Effective Renal Plasma Flow (ERPF).—

Normal Value.—633 ml./min./1·73 sq. m. body surface-area.

If a substance is completely removed from the plasma during one passage through the kidneys, then its excretion rate measures the renal plasma flow. Para-aminohippurate and diodone in low plasma concentrations are approximately 90 per cent extracted and therefore can be used to measure the effective renal plasma flow.

Then,

$$\frac{\text{Glomerular Filtration Rate (GFR)}}{\text{Effective Renal Plasma Flow (ERPF)}}$$
$$= \text{Filtration Fraction (FF)}$$
$$= 0 \cdot 2 \text{ approximately.}$$

In the presence of renal tubular damage, the arteriovenous difference in concentration of para-aminohippurate or of diodone must be known before the ERPF can be calculated.

Filtration Fraction.—

Increase in the filtration fraction is supposed to indicate increased constrictor tone in the glomerular efferent arterioles.

Decrease in the filtration fraction implies that the glomerular filtration rate is reduced.

The measurement of these various fractions is probably only justified in the investigation of certain cases in specialized units.

GLUCAGON IN PLASMA

Normal Range.—0·4–1·4 ng./ml.

The bioassay depends on the measurement of lipolysis of isolated chicken fat cells.

REFERENCE.—Langslow, D. R., and Hales, C. N. (1970), *Lancet*, 1, 1151.

Pathological.—

Increase.—Acute pancreatitis.

GLUCAGON TOLERANCE TEST

After a diet unrestricted in carbohydrates for at least 3 days and after an overnight fast, an initial fasting blood-glucose sample is taken. One milligram of glucagon is injected intramuscularly (in children 30 μg./kg. body-weight up to a maximum dose of 1 mg.). Blood-glucose samples are taken at 15 minutes, 30 minutes, and then every ½ hour for a total of 3 hours.

Normal Result.—There is a rapid rise in blood-glucose by not less than 40 mg./100 ml. at 15–30 minutes, and by 30–90 mg./100 ml. at ½–1 hour, returning to near the fasting blood-glucose level by 3 hours. Reactive hypoglycæmia does not occur.

Pathological.—

1. Normal or greater than normal hyperglycæmia response which is rapidly followed by severe hypoglycæmia.
   a. Pancreatic islet-cell tumour (insulinoma).
   b. Idiopathic hypoglycæmia in children.
2. Absence or grossly reduced initial hyperglycæmia.—
   a. Liver glycogen storage disease. (Types I, III, and glycogen synthetase deficiency. Abnormally small increases in blood-glucose occur in Types IV, V, and VI.)
   b. Hypoglycæmia due to liver damage.
   c. Hypoglycæmia due to endocrine disorders, e.g., hypoadrenalism, hypopituitarism.
   d. Hypoglycæmia due to malnutrition.

This is a useful screening test for islet-cell tumours of the pancreas and for idiopathic hypoglycæmia in children. It is important to have intravenous glucose solution and adrenaline available in case the induced hypoglycæmia is severe.

REFERENCE.—Marks, V., and Rose, F. C. (1965), *Hypoglycæmia*. Oxford: Blackwell.

GLUCOSE (Sugar)

The body glucose pool is mainly in the extracellular fluid and the liver intracellular fluid, and consists of 10–20 g. glucose in a normal adult. The circulating glucose has a half-life of 40 minutes ($\equiv$ 200 mg. turned over every minute).

GLUCOSE IN BLOOD (Fasting).—

Normal Range. (As true glucose):—
1. Venous blood: 45–95 mg./100 ml. (2·5–5·3 mmol./litre). As true glucose.
2. Arterial and capillary blood: 50–90 mg./100 ml. (2·8–5·0 mmol./litre). As true glucose.

$$\left(\frac{\text{mg./litre}}{180} = \text{mmol./litre.} \right)$$

3. Normal total blood-"sugar"=up to 20 mg./100 ml. higher than (1) or (2). (Many methods estimate glucose+non-glucose reducing substances.)

Physiological.—
Increase in Fasting Level.—Due to increased circulating adrenaline:—
1. Strenuous exercise.
2. Strong emotion, e.g., fear.
Decrease in Fasting Level.—
1. Mild hypoglycæmia has been reported in normal pregnancy.
2. Severe hypoglycæmia occurs in normal newborn infants of diabetic mothers.
3. At birth the blood-glucose falls to its lowest level at 2–4 hours, regaining the birth level by 3–5 days.

Pathological.—
Increase.—
1. *Increased Circulating Adrenaline.*—
   a. After injection of adrenaline.
   b. Shock.
   c. Phæochromocytoma, in an attack.
   d. Possibly in severe thyrotoxicosis.
   e. Burns. Hyperglycæmia occurs for a few hours to days after a burn.
2. *Diabetes Mellitus.*—
   a. Insulin deficient type.
   b. Insulin resistant type.
3. *Pituitary and Adrenal Disorders.*—
   a. Cushing's syndrome. This condition is frequently complicated by an insulin resistant diabetes.
   b. Gigantism and acromegaly. In the early stages there is an insulin resistant diabetes. Hypopituitarism develops later.

c. Following ACTH injections 11-oxysteroids are released, leading to increased gluconeogenesis and also inhibition of carbohydrate utilization.

4. *Pancreatic Disease.*—

    a. Acute (and some cases of chronic) pancreatitis.

    b. Rarely in extensive pancreatic carcinoma.

5. *Vitamin-B_1 Deficiency.*—Wernicke's encephalopathy.

6. Hyperglycæmia during peritoneal dialysis or hæmodialysis appears to be associated with hypokalæmia.

REFERENCE.—Seedat, Y. K. (1968), *Lancet*, 2, 1166.

In hyperglycæmic states glucose exerts an osmotic pressure which expands the extracellular space at the expense of the intracellular space. Every 100 mg./100 ml. increase in blood glucose above a basal blood glucose of 100 mg./100 ml. causes a reduction in plasma sodium of about 3 mEq./litre (by dilution). This should be remembered during intravenous fluid therapy.

Decrease.—

1. *Insulin Excess.*—

    a. Pancreatic islet cell:—

        i. Hyperplasia.

        ii. Adenoma.

        iii. Carcinoma.

    b. Insulin overdosage, e.g., "missed meal" in a diabetic.

    c. Post-gastrectomy dumping syndrome. Rapid absorption of carbohydrate by small intestine leads to release of insulin which continues to act after most of the carbohydrate has been absorbed and stored.

    d. Functional hypoglycæmia. Probably there is excessively rapid absorption as in (c).

    e. Hypothalamic lesions. These may cause vagal stimulation of the pancreatic islet cells but this is rare,

2. *Insulin Antagonist Deficiency.*—

    a. Adrenal cortical insufficiency (Addison's disease).

    b. Hypopituitarism.

3. *Deficiency in Available Glycogen.*—

    a. *Liver Disease.*—

        i. Acute infections.—

            α. Viral hepatitis (rare).

            β. Yellow fever.

        ii. Poisons.—

            α. Organic arsenic.

            β. Carbon tetrachloride.

            γ. Chloroform.

            δ. Cinchophen.

            ε. Phosphorus.

            ζ. Alcohol.

            η. Acute paracetamol poisoning.

        iii. Terminal cirrhosis of the liver (some cases).

        iv. Multiple hepatic carcinomatous deposits (rare).

        v. Von Gierke's liver glycogen storage disease.

    b. *Renal Glycosuria.*—(Very uncommon cause.)

4. *Immaturity.*—Neonatal hypoglycæmia may occur particularly in—

    a. Underweight, poorly nourished babies.

 b. Twins.

 c. Premature infants.

 d. Infants of diabetic mothers.

 Glucose apparently passes abnormally rapidly into the cells, since the cell membranes are incompletely developed. The serum calcium level may also fall.

N.B.—In diabetes mellitus after prolonged hyperglycæmia, and subsequent treatment with insulin, symptoms of hypoglycæmia occur at a higher blood-sugar level than normal.

 Hypoglycæmia in Children.—

  1. *Organic.*—

   a. Islet cell tumour of the pancreas.

   b. Hypopituitarism.

   c. Addison's disease.

   d. Severe liver disease.

   e. Galactosæmia. Following ingestion of galactose, blood glucose falls (as blood galactose rises) to dangerously low levels.

   f. Hereditary fructose intolerance after oral fructose.

   g. Kwashiorkor.

  2. *Functional.*—

   a. Occurs in nervous, highly strung, children. Fasting blood-sugar normal, glucose tolerance curve normal but followed by hypoglycæmia at 2–3 hours. (Patient must be on high carbohydrate diet for some days before test.) The condition gradually remits.

   b. Occurs in infants, and presents with convulsions. There is a real danger of brain damage caused by hypoglycæmia. Daily ACTH prevents hypoglycæmia, and the condition gradually remits. Pituitary and adrenal function is normal, and liver glycogen stores are normal.

REFERENCES.—Editorial (1954), *Lancet*, 2, 276; Editorial (1959), *Ibid.*, 2, 500 (endogenous hypoglycæmia); Marks, V., and Rose, F. C. (1965), *Hypoglycæmia.* Oxford: Blackwell.

GLUCOSE IN CEREBROSPINAL FLUID.—

Normal Range.—

 In cisternal and lumbar fluid the glucose concentration is about 10–20 mg./100 ml. less than the blood concentration. The ventricular fluid glucose is more nearly approximate to the blood-glucose level.

Pathological.—

 Increase.—

  1. Diabetic hyperglycæmia.

  2. Epidemic encephalitis.

  3. Syphilis of the central nervous system (slight increase).

 Decrease.—

  1. Infection (meningitis).—

   a. Bacteria:—

    i. Suppurative.

    ii. Tuberculous.

   b. Fungi.

   c. Viruses. Mumps meningo-encephalitis, associated with CSF glucose <40 mg. per cent, persistent pleocytosis, and raised protein.

2. Other conditions with gross pleocytosis (e.g., syphilitic meningitis).
3. Multiple tumours in the meninges, but these are rare causes:—
   a. Carcinoma.
   b. Sarcoma.
   c. Lymphoma.
4. Sarcoidosis involving the central nervous system.
5. Hypoglycæmia. (*See* GLUCOSE IN BLOOD for possible causes.)

N.B.—The cerebrospinal fluid glucose may be normal in viral infections, and may be normal in tuberculous meningitis. Further observations with parallel blood-sugar estimations are required in poliomyelitis, lymphocytic meningitis, and viral encephalitis.

REFERENCES.—Wilfert, Catherine M. (1969), *New Engl. J. Med.*, **280**, 855; Gaines, J. D., Eckman, P. B., and Remington, J. S. (1970), *Arch. Intern. Med.*, **125**, 333.

GLUCOSE IN PLEURAL EFFUSION.—The finding of low glucose concentrations in pleural effusions has not been of diagnostic value.

REFERENCE.—Glenert, J. (1962), *Acta Tuberc. pneumologica scand.*, **42**, 22.

GLUCOSE TOLERANCE TEST.—The patient must be on a full mixed diet for at least three days, preferably for seven days, before the test is performed.

After starvation or a low carbohydrate diet, tolerance is diminished and a normal person will have a blood-sugar peak during the test of more than 200 mg./100 ml.

The patient must fast overnight. Excitement, fear, exercise, and unaccustomed or excessive tobacco smoking may diminish tolerance. It appears that glucose tolerance in non-obese subjects is related both to insulin sensitivity and insulin release.

REFERENCE.—Martin, F. I. R., Pearson, M. J., and Stocks, A. E. (1968), *Lancet*, **1**, 1285.

INTRAVENOUS TEST.—Glucose, 0·5 g./kg. body-weight as an aqueous 20 per cent solution, is injected intravenously over a period of 30 minutes. After a normal fasting level, a peak blood-sugar of 200–250 mg./100 ml. is reached immediately. The fasting level is regained by 90 minutes, and sub-fasting levels occur at 2 hours, returning to the fasting level by 3 hours. Because of the high blood-sugar levels attained, some glycosuria is normal.

1. In liver disease, because of inability to form glycogen rapidly, the fall from the peak values is delayed, fasting levels being regained by 3–5 hours. Results with the oral glucose tolerance test in liver disease are variable.
2. In Addison's disease and hypopituitarism the peak levels are normal (cf. flattened curve in oral test) but severe hypoglycæmia follows.
3. In hypothyroidism the test is normal, cf. oral test.
4. Defective intestinal absorption of glucose, cf. flat oral curve.

In cases of glucose-6-phosphate dehydrogenase deficiency, although the oral test is normal significantly higher results are obtained with the intravenous test.

N.B.—Generally the oral glucose tolerance test is most useful in the diagnosis of diabetes mellitus, and, when the test is prolonged, in the diagnosis of excessive pancreatic islet cell activity.

As glucose tolerance decreases, so also the arteriovenous (capillary-venous) blood-sugar difference decreases and vice versa. The 1-hour 2-dose test is not normally performed in this country.

REFERENCES.—Exton, W. G., and Rose, A. R. (1934), *Amer. J. clin. Path.*, **4**, 381; Ross, C. W., and Tonks, E. L. (1938), *Arch. Dis. Childh.*, **13**, 289.

ORAL TEST.—
Method.—
1. Adults—50 g. glucose in 100 ml. of water (or 1·0 g./kg. body-weight).
2. Children up to 8 years old—20 g. glucose in water.
3. Children 8–12 years old—30 g. glucose in water.
4. 14–15 years old—40 g. glucose in water.

N.B.—The maximum response is obtained in children using 1·75 g./kg. body-weight.

Within limits the rate of absorption of glucose from the intestine is fairly constant although there is a diurnal variation, higher results being found in the afternoon.

Blood Samples are collected at 0, 30, 60, 90, 120, 150, and 180 minutes. Arterial and capillary samples tend to give higher readings than venous samples. This difference reflects the degree of glucose utilization. The difference averages about 30 mg./100 ml. Urine samples are collected hourly. Plasma potassium and inorganic phosphate levels both reciprocate the blood-glucose curve, since both potassium and phosphate enter the body cells from the extracellular fluid.

Results.—
Normal.—
1. *Normal Fasting Level.*—This should be less than 100 mg./100 ml. as true glucose (or less than 120 mg./100 ml. as total sugar).
2. *Normal Peak.*—The peak reaches 160–180 mg./100 ml. by ½–1 hr.
3. Normal fasting level is regained in 2 hours.
4. *Normal Subsequent Temporary Sub-fasting Level.*—The blood-sugar falls to 10–15 mg./100 ml. less than the fasting level. This fall is proportional to the height and rapidity of rise of the peak of the curve. It depends directly on the amount of glucose given and the rapidity of its absorption.

Pathological.—
1. Diminished Tolerance.—
   a. *Fasting Hyperglycæmia.*—*See* possible causes under GLUCOSE IN BLOOD.
   b. *Excessive Height of Peak.*—
      i. *Increased Rate of Absorption from Intestine.*—
         α. "Alimentary". Excessive glucose intake.
         β. Hyperthyroidism. There is an early high peak and then a rapid fall in blood-sugar to normal.

γ. Postgastrectomy, gastro-enterostomy, and vagotomy. The blood-sugar rises to a high early peak and then falls rapidly to below the fasting level. The period of hypoglycæmia may be prolonged, and is probably due to excessive production of insulin in response to the very rapid rate of glucose absorption.

δ. "Lag" curve. As (γ), but there is no previous gastrectomy or gastro-enterostomy.

ii. *Increased Glycogenolysis and Gluconeogenesis.*—

α. Hyperthyroidism.

β. Hyperadrenalism, due to strong emotion, or phæochromocytoma.

γ. Toxæmia associated with infections.

δ. Pregnancy. There is a mild decrease in tolerance, particularly in the third trimester.

iii. *Inability to form Glycogen from Administered Glucose.*—

α. Severe liver damage.

β. Von Gierke's liver glycogen storage disease.
In both these conditions, the fasting level is low and the test is followed by hypoglycæmia.

iv. *Inability of Tissues to utilize Glucose.*—

α. Diabetes mellitus.

β. Hæmochromatosis with associated diabetes mellitus.

γ. "Steroid diabetes", caused by Cushing's syndrome, ACTH administration, or adrenal cortical steroid administration, e.g., hydrocortisone.

δ. Head injury and intracranial lesions may be associated with damage to, or pressure in, the hypothalamic region.

ε. Following insulin shock therapy.

The blood-sugar concentration rises to abnormally high levels, remaining raised, and falling towards the fasting level slowly, in this group (iv), α, β, γ, and δ.

c. *Return to the Fasting Blood-sugar Level.*—In the conditions listed in (i) and (ii), the fasting level is regained within 3 hours. In diabetes mellitus and "steroid diabetes" (*see* iv), the fasting level is frequently abnormally raised, and is not regained for some hours after glucose.

d. *Associated Glycosuria.*—In the presence of normal renal tubular function, filtered glucose is completely reabsorbed, until the blood-sugar level reaches approximately 160 mg./100 ml. (The critical concentration, or threshold, varies with the rate of urine flow.)

i. *Alimentary Glycosuria.*—The fasting urine is free of sugar, and at least the final urine specimen contains sugar.

ii. *Diabetic Glycosuria.*—As (i), unless the fasting blood-sugar exceeds the renal threshold for glucose, when sugar will be found in all specimens.

N.B.—**In diabetes mellitus the renal threshold for glucose rises.**

iii. *Renal Glycosuria.*—Sugar appears in the urine even when the blood-sugar level is below the normal renal threshold.

2. Increased Tolerance.—

    a. Fasting Hypoglycæmia.—*See* possible causes under GLUCOSE IN BLOOD. To demonstrate true hypoglycæmia use:—

        i. Arterial or freely flowing capillary blood.

        ii. True glucose estimation method.

    b. Flattened Blood-sugar Peak.—

        i. *Poor Rate of Absorption from Intestine.*—

          α. Hypoadrenalism (Addison's disease).

          β. Hypopituitarism, with secondary hypoadrenalism.

          γ. Intestinal disease, including steatorrhœa (i.e., cœliac disease, idiopathic steatorrhœa, or sprue, tuberculous enteritis, and Whipple's disease).

          δ. Hypothyroidism.

        ii. *Excessive Insulin Secretion.*—

          α. Hyperplasia of pancreatic islet cells, e.g., after prolonged excessive carbohydrate intake.

          β. Pancreatic islet cell adenoma.

          γ. Pancreatic islet cell carcinoma.

        iii. *Exaggerated Hypoglycæmic Phase.*—After the return of the blood-sugar to the fasting level, it may fall by a further 20 mg./100 ml. or more and remain low for 1 hour or more, with symptoms of hypoglycæmia. This occurs particularly with islet cell hyperplasia, adenoma, carcinoma, or chronic pancreatitis. Where these conditions are suspected, a prolonged glucose tolerance test lasting up to 8 hours may reveal such a severe hypoglycæmic phase. This will also occur in hypopituitarism and liver disease.

REFERENCES.—Boyns, D. R., Crossley, J. N., Abrams, M. F., Jarrett, R. J., and Keen, H. (1969), *Brit. med. J.*, 1, 595, 599; Hunter, R., Jones, Muriel, Hurn, B. A. L., and Duncan, Catherine (1970), *Ibid.*, 1, 465.

URINE SUGAR.—
1. GLUCOSE.—
Normal Output.—1–15 mg./100 ml.

    Glycosuria.—

        1. *Renal Glycosuria.*—

          a. Congenital renal defect.

          b. Very rarely in acute renal failure.

          c. Phlorizin poisoning.

        2. *Rapid Intestinal Absorption.*—

          a. "Lag" glycosuria.

          b. Postgastrectomy glycosuria (dumping syndrome).

          c. In normal pregnancy there may be unduly rapid absorption from the intestine.

        3. *Ductless Gland Disorders.*—

          a. Pancreas. Diabetes mellitus.

          b. Thyroid. Thyrotoxicosis.

    c. Pituitary:—
        i. Gigantism.
        ii. Acromegaly.
        iii. Cushing's syndrome.
    d. Adrenal. Adrenal cortical hyperplasia.
4. *Sepsis* (glucose tolerance diminished).
5. Head injury cases and some cases of intracranial tumour. Related to hypothalamic pressure or damage.
6. Massive oral glucose intake, especially after a poor diet (vagabond's glycosuria).
7. *Wernicke's encephalopathy* (some cases).
8. Glycosuria frequent in lead poisoning in infants and children.

REFERENCE.—Fine, J. (1965), *Brit. med. J.*, 1, 1209.

2. LACTOSE.—Occurs particularly in the afternoon:—
1. Late pregnancy in normal women.
2. During normal lactation in women.
3. Alactasia after ingestion of lactose in diet.

3. GALACTOSE.—
1. After galactose tolerance in normal individuals.
2. Liver disease (some cases).
3. Galactosæmia.

4. LÆVULOSE.—
1. Alimentary (especially associated with liver disease). After ingestion of honey and grapes.
2. Essential fructosuria. An inborn error of metabolism of no clinical importance.
3. Fructose intolerance. Excessive rise in blood lævulose and excessive fall in blood glucose after oral lævulose.

5. PENTOSE.—
1. Alimentary (e.g., cherries and plums in excess).
2. Alleged to appear in a few cases of diabetes mellitus (severe).
3. Essential pentosuria. A familial hereditary condition occurring mainly in Jewish males.

REFERENCE.—Touster, O. (1959), *Amer. J. Med.*, 26, 724 (141 references).

6. RIBOSURIA.—In this form of pentosuria, which is associated with muscular dystrophy, the ribose is probably derived from the nucleoprotein of breaking down muscle-cells, as in progressive muscular atrophy.

7. SUCROSURIA.—
1. Benign. Occurs in the newborn on an artificial diet.
2. Non-benign. It is associated with infants with mental defect, raised plasma potassium concentrations, and hiatus hernia.
3. May occur in association with pancreatic disease.
4. Artefact.

8. 'NON-SUGARS' WHICH REDUCE BENEDICT'S RE-AGENT.—
1. Urine, which has a high concentration of uric acid or creatinine.

2. Glycuronates. Salicylates are excreted as glycuronates. After therapeutic doses of para-aminosalicylates (PAS) there is an apparent glycosuria.
3. Formaldehyde. Appears in the urine after methyl alcohol ingestion.
4. Homogentisic acid.
5. Phenylpyruvic acid.

Paper chromatography is a very useful method for the identification of sugars and "sugar-like" substances in the urine.

GLUTEN TOLERANCE TEST

After 700 mg. gluten per kg. body-weight, by mouth, the blood glutamine level in cases of cœliac disease rises to three times the normal increase. Unfortunately there is a wide overlap of results in controls and coeliac cases.

REFERENCES.—Alvey, C., Anderson, C. M., and Freeman, M. (1957), *Arch. Dis. Childh.*, **32**, 434; Payne, W. W., and Jenkinson, V (1958), *Ibid.*, **33**, 413.

GONADOTROPHINS IN URINE

1. HUMAN CHORIONIC GONADOTROPHIN (HCG).—Synthesized by normal or malignant trophoblast cells, this glycoprotein, with a probable molecular weight of 26,000–30,000, can be detected and estimated in the urine.

Physiological.—In normal pregnancy chorionic gonadotrophins can be detected by the end of the 6th week. Peak values occur between the 12th and 16th weeks, disappearing after delivery, pregnancy tests becoming negative by the ninth day. Higher levels are found in multiple pregnancies.

Pathological.—
Increase.—
    1. Hydatidiform mole. A rising titre at the end of the first trimester is significant. Titres can rise to 1000 i.u./ml. or more.
    2. Choriocarcinoma of uterus.
    3. Choriocarcinoma of testis.
Decrease.—
    1. Ectopic pregnancy. Low values for the stage of pregnancy.
    2. Inevitable or threatened abortion. Low values for the stage of pregnancy. Low values in early pregnancy are found in habitual abortion.
    3. Following total hysterectomy for hydatidiform mole, the very high output of HCG falls within 24 hours, reaching 1 i.u./ml. by the seventh to eleventh days post-operation. If the titre remains in the urine for several weeks after operation, this suggests involvement of deeper uterine involvement, following surgical removal of hydatidiform mole.

2. HUMAN PITUITARY GONADOTROPHINS (FOLLICULAR STIMULATING HORMONE, FSH).—
Physiological.—Low levels are normally found in children.

Pathological.—

Increased.—

1. Seminoma of the testis.
2. Klinefelter's syndrome.
3. Turner's syndrome.
4. Ovarian amenorrhœa.
5. Castration.
6. Corticosteroid therapy.

Decreased.—

1. Œstrogen therapy.
2. Progesterone therapy.

3. HUMAN LUTEINIZING HORMONE (LH).—Mid-cycle ovulatory values are two to six times higher than non-ovulatory values.

Post-menopausal values in women are two to ten times higher than non-ovulatory values.

GROWTH HORMONE IN SERUM

Following the action of growth-hormone releasing factor from the hypothalamus on the pituitary, growth hormone (HGH) is released in intermittent bursts. It consists of a polypeptide containing 188 amino-acid residues, with a molecular weight of 27,000, and with a half-life of approximately 20 minutes, diurnal variation, with highest levels occurring during sleep.

Growth hormone stimulates production of messenger-RNA and causes proliferation of epiphysial cartilage cells, and diminishes sensitivity to insulin.

Normal Values.—0–7·7 ng./ml.

Physiological.—

Increase.—

During normal pregnancy in both mother and fœtus.
After overnight fast.
After carbohydrate-rich meal.
After exercise.
Anxiety.
Œstrogens and androgens increase HGH and enhance responsiveness.

Pathological.—

Increase.—

Acute illness.
Trauma, surgery.
Acromegaly.
Gigantism.
Hypoglycæmia.

Decrease.—

Panhypopituitarism.
Pituitary dwarfism.

A. AFTER INSULIN-INDUCED HYPOGLYCÆMIA (0·1 unit/kg. body-weight i.v.; 0·05 unit/kg. body-weight i.v. in children).—

Normal serum levels rise to 15–121 ng./ml. at 30–60 minutes.

Pathological Response.—

No increase.—

Hypopituitarism (hypoglycæmia may be dangerous).
Hypothyroidism (especially in children).

Hyperadrenocorticalism.

Corticosteroid suppression in adults.

Some otherwise normal obese subjects show only a small rise in growth hormone following hypoglycæmia.

B. AFTER 100 g. ORAL GLUCOSE.—

1 Hour:

Normal.—Serum growth hormone levels fall to less than 1 ng./ml.

Pathological Response.—

No decrease in serum growth hormone.—Acromegaly. This is a very good test for the detection of acromegaly, but is not useful to define the severity of the condition.

4 Hours later: The normal serum growth hormone level rises. This is a useful test of the ability of children to secrete growth hormone.

C. AFTER ARGININE INFUSION (0·5 g./kg. body-weight over 30 minutes).—

Normal.—The serum growth hormone level rises by more than 10 ng./ml.

Pathological Response.—There is no response in pituitary dwarfs.

D. AFTER GLUCAGON INJECTION.—Blood samples are taken at 0, 60, 120, 150, and 180 min. after 1 mg. glucagon i.m. or subcut. (1·5 mg. for subjects over 90 kg.).

Normal.—

Females.—Mean fasting values of up to 7·1 ng./ml. Mean peak values of 20·3 ng./ml.

Males.—Mean fasting values of up to 3·7 ng./ml. Mean peak values of 18·8 ng./ml.

Pathological.—Peak values of less than 7 ng./ml. = deficiency of HGH.

The pattern of response to insulin-induced hypoglycæmia, arginine infusion, basal serum growth hormone estimation, and response to exogenous growth hormone has been used successfully to classify sexual atleiotic dwarfism.

Acute metabolic response to injected human growth hormone is greatest in those patients with no measurable serum growth hormone response to insulin-induced hypoglycæmia.

Arginine monochloride is expensive, and male subjects require 1–2 days of œstrogen therapy before response is obtainable.

REFERENCES.—Schalch, D. S., and Parker, M. L. (1964), *Nature, Lond.*, **203**, 1141; Lazarus, L., and Young, J. D. (1966), *J. clin. Endocrin.*, **26**, 213; Melvin, K. E. W., Wright, A. D., Hartog, M., Artcliff, A. C., Copestake, A. M., and Russell Fraser, T. (1967), *Brit. med. J.*, **3**, 196; Goodman, H. G., Grumbach, M. M., and Kaplan, Selna L. (1968), *New Engl. J. Med.*, **278**, 57; Merimee, T. J., Hall, J. D., Rimoin, D. L., and McKusick, V. A. (1969), *Lancet*, **1**, 963; Catt, K. J. (1970), *Ibid.*, **1**, 933; Mitchell, M. L., Byrne, M. J., Sanchez, Y., and Sawin, C. T. (1970), *New Engl. J. Med.*, **282**, 539.

HÆMOGLOBIN IN PLASMA*

Normal Range.—1–4 mg./100 ml.

Pathological.—

Increase.—

    1. Marked increase (intravascular hæmolysis), e.g.:—

       a. Paroxysmal nocturnal hæmoglobinuria.

* *See also* HAPTOGLOBINS (p. 144) and METHÆMALBUMIN (p. 102).

      b. Cold hæmoglobinuria.
      c. Blackwater fever.
  2. Moderate increase:—
      a. Acquired hæmolytic anæmia.
      b. Sickle-cell anæmia.
      c. Thalassæmia major.

N.B.—No increase occurs in hereditary spherocytosis, since red-cell breakdown occurs extravascularly in the spleen.

It is important to avoid hæmolysis during or after collection of the blood sample, or the result is invalid.

HIPPURIC ACID EXCRETION TEST

The normal liver conjugates glycine with benzoic acid to form hippuric acid. This probably occurs in two stages. Since the liver synthesizes glycine, a load in the form of sodium benzoate should measure:—

  1. Rate of synthesis of glycine by the liver.
  2. Rate of formation of hippuric acid by the liver.

ORAL TEST.—6 g. sodium benzoate orally should result in the excretion of 4·4 g. $\pm$ 15 per cent hippuric acid in the urine within 4 hours in a normal person.

INTRAVENOUS TEST.—1·77 g. sodium benzoate is injected intravenously. This should result in an excretion of 0·7–0·95 g. hippuric acid in the urine in 1 hour in a normal person.

N.B.—**There appears to be a greater norma variation after the intravenous test.**

Pathological.—

  Decrease.—
    1. *Liver Damage.*—
      a. Hepatitis.
      b. Cirrhosis (both portal and biliary types).
      c. Secondary carcinoma infiltrating the liver.
      d. Hepatic necrosis.
      e. Obstructive jaundice, if the obstruction is prolonged.
    2. *Renal Damage.*—Renal tubule excretion of hippurate is diminished in nephritis and nephrosclerosis.
    3. *Hepatic and Renal Impairment.*—Congestive cardiac failure.
    4. *Possible Protein Deficiency.*—
      a. Cachexia   { Possibly associated with poor
      b. Chronic anæmia   glycine formation, and some
                               tubule damage.

N.B.—The excretion of hippuric acid in any patient varies with the rate of urine-flow. It has been suggested that after 3 g. oral para-aminobenzoic acid, the blood para-aminohippuric acid level at 1 hour measures liver function. A low blood-level indicates liver damage.

REFERENCE.—Deiss, W. P., and Cohen, P. P. (1950), *J. clin. Invest.*, 29, 1014.

17-HYDROXYCORTICOIDS IN URINE

The estimation of 17-hydroxycorticoids includes cortisone, hydrocortisone, and their metabolites. Moxham and Nabarro

(1956) found good correlation between the urinary output of 17-hydroxycorticoids and 17-oxogenic steroids.

Normal Urine Output in Adults.—

Males—108–396 μg./24 hr.

Females—78–311 μg./24 hr.

The output is increased in late normal pregnancy.

The ratio of 11-deoxy-17-oxosteroids to 17-hydroxycortico-steroids has not been found to be of prognostic value in carcinoma of the breast.

After Corticotrophin Gel.—

1. *No Increase in Output.*—

   a. Addison's disease, untreated.

   b. Addison's disease, treated with cortisone. The daily output of urine 17-hydroxycorticosteroids is normal (derived from administered cortisone), but there is no response to ACTH.

2. *Increased Output.*—

   a. Hypopituitarism (the adrenal cortex can respond).

   b. Cushing's syndrome. The control levels are above normal, and there is marked response to ACTH.

   c. During long-term treatment of rheumatoid arthritis with ACTH it has been found that clinical improvement occurs when the urine 17-hydroxycorticoid excretion increases by 50 per cent.

   d. Early stages of mountain sickness.

REFERENCES.—Moxham, A., and Nabarro, J. D. N. (1956), *J. clin. Path.*, **9**, 351; Savage, O., Chapman, L., Robertson, J. D., Davis, P., Popert, A. J., and Copeman, W. S. C. (1957), *Brit. med. J.*, **2**, 1257; Jenkins, J. S. (1958), *J. clin. Path.*, **11**, 78; *Lancet* (1963), **1**, 1415, Medical Research Council recommendations.

11-HYDROXYCORTICOSTEROIDS IN PLASMA
(Approximately equal to plasma cortisol)

Normal Range.—

(Most of the cortisol is protein-bound. Only the free portion is metabolically active. When plasma cortisol exceeds 20–25 μg./100 ml. the protein is saturated.)

Sample at 9 a.m.=8–26 μg./100 ml. ($14\pm3\cdot5$ μg./100 ml.).

Sample at 4 p.m.=2–18 μg./100 ml.

Sample at midnight=less than 6 μg./100 ml. ($5\pm1\cdot5$ μg./100 ml.).

Levels increased during normal pregnancy. Also plasma cortisol increases after intravenous fructose.

Pathological.—

Diurnal Rhythm.—

Raised levels without loss of rhythm:—

   1. Stress, including fever, severe pain.

   2. Some cases of Cushing's syndrome.

Loss of diurnal rhythm with no evening decrease:—

   1. Acute infections.

   2. Encephalitis.

   3. Central nervous system tumours, with raised intra-cranial pressure.

   4. Acromegaly.

   5. Carcinomatosis.

6. Congestive cardiac failure.
7. Liver damage.
8. Renovascular hypertension.
9. Pituitary hyperactivity.

Increase.—

1. Cushing's syndrome.
2. Hypothyroidism ⎤
3. Liver disease   ⎟ Due to slow disposal of circulating
4. Terminal states ⎦ cortisol.
5. Œstrogen therapy, due to increased level of circulating specific plasma cortisol-binding protein (as in normal pregnancy).
6. Accidental hypothermia (may rise above 30 μg./100 ml.).
7. Early stages of mountain sickness.
8. Alcohol excess in non-alcoholics. No rise in chronic alcoholics.
9. After amphetamine.
10. Some psychotics.

Decrease.—

1. Addison's disease, with primary failure of the adrenal cortex.
2. Hypopituitarism, with secondary failure of the adrenal cortex.
3. Adrenal pituitary suppression following long-term ACTH or steroid therapy may be detected by inadequate rise in plasma cortisol following insulin-induced hypoglycæmia.

    In severe infection with hypotension plasma levels of less than 15 μg./100 ml. = inadequate adrenal cortical response.

REFERENCES.—Mattingly, D. (1962), *J. clin. Path.*, **15**, 374; Jacobs, H. S., and Nabarro, J. D. N. (1963), *Brit. med. J.*, **2**, 595; Merry, J., and Marks, V. (1969), *Lancet*, **1**, 921; Carter, Mary E., and James, V. H. T. (1970), *Ibid.*, **1**, 328; Sprunt, J. G., Maclean, D., and Browning, M. C. K. (1970), *Ibid.*, **1**, 324.

A rapid test for adrenocortical insufficiency may be performed by taking an initial blood-sample for cortisol estimation, followed by intramuscular injection of 25 units of ACTH. A second blood-sample is taken after 1 hour.

Normal controls: Plasma cortisol increased by +24·7 μg./100 ml. (+11·3 to +47·8 μg./100 ml. plasma).
Adrenocortical failure (Addison's disease): Plasma cortisol increased by 0·5 μg./100 ml. (−1·5 to +2·6 μg./100 ml. plasma).
Aldactone interferes with the estimation of plasma cortisol.

REFERENCE.—Maynard, D. E., Folk, R. L., Riley, T. R., Wieland, R. G., Gwinup, G., and Hamwi, G. J. (1966), *Ann. intern. Med.*, **65**, 552.

11-HYDROXYCORTICOSTEROIDS IN URINE

Normal Range.—
Adult males—108–396 μg./24 hr.
Adult females—75–307 μg./24 hr.
Plasma cortisol estimation is to be preferred.

5-HYDROXYINDOLACETIC ACID IN URINE

5-hydroxyindolacetic acid is a metabolite of 5-hydroxy-tryptamine (serotonin, enteramine). The normal range of excretion of 5-hydroxyindolacetic acid is 3–14 mg./24 hr.

Pathological.—

Increase.—

1. *Carcinoid Tumours.—*The urine output varies from 40 to 2000 μg./24 hr. Where the carcinoid tumour is successfully removed the urine excretion drops to normal. If the tumour is incompletely removed, or if secondary deposits remain, the urine excretion remains abnormal.
2. *Alimentary Carcinoma.—*There may be a slight increase above normal output in some cases.
3. *Pulmonary Carcinoma.—*Oat-cell carcinoma of the bronchus and bronchial adenoma of carcinoid type may secrete excess 5-hydroxyindolacetic acid.

Decrease—

*Mastocytosis.—*5-hydroxyindolacetic acid is absent from the urine.

REFERENCES.—Jepson, J. B. (1955), *Lancet*, **2**, 1009. (This paper describes the technique of paper chromatography applied to the urine indoles.); Snow, P. J. D., Lennard-Jones, J. E., Curzon, G., and Stacey, R. S. (1955), *Ibid.*, **2**, 1004.

N.B.—It has been reported that a high banana diet results in increased urine 5-hydroxyindolacetic acid excretion, and that some cases of idiopathic steatorrhœa also show an increased 5-hydroxyindolacetic acid excretion. Mephesin and acetanilide give false positive colour reactions, whilst chlorpromazine and other phenothiazine derivatives have a quenching effect on colour production during the estimation.

REFERENCES.—Report from American Gastro-enterological Association (1958), *Lancet*, **1**, 1313; Editorial (1964), *Brit. med. J.*, **1**, 6; Gowenlock, A. H., Platt, D. S., Campbell, A. C. P., and Wormsley, K. G. (1964), *Lancet*, **1**, 304.

4-HYDROXY-3-METHOXY-MANDELIC ACID

See Catecholamines

HYDROXYPROLINE (TOTAL) IN URINE

Normal Range.—In adults the output is 6–42 mg./g. creatinine, up to 55 years of age. In old age the output increases with increased natural breakdown of collagen and reduced creatinine excretion (related to decrease in muscle mass). Collagen is rich in hydroxyproline. There is a diurnal rhythm of excretion with greater excretion overnight.

Excess excretion of free hydroxyproline occurs in a specific inborn error of metabolism, in various non-specific amino-acidurias, and in amino-aciduria associated with bone dystrophy. Otherwise hydroxyproline is excreted as peptide complexes, requiring hydrolysis before estimation.

Pathological.—

Increase.—

1. Any condition with increased bone turnover.
2. Thyrotoxicosis.

3. Increased parathyroid hormone activity.
4. Hydroxyprolinæmia (rare).
5. Osteomalacia after vitamin D.

Decrease.—
1. Dwarfs (bone contains 40 per cent of the total body collagen).
2. Following calcium infusion.

REFERENCE.—Smith, R., and Dick, M. (1968), *Lancet*, 1, 279.

INSULIN IN SERUM

FASTING LEVELS.—
Physiological.—
*Normal Values.—*4–30 μU./ml. (mean=17 μU./ml.). (Serum is preferred to plasma since heparin affects the results obtained in plasma.)
Increased.—
1. Some otherwise normal obese subjects.
2. Normal pregnancy.
3. Fructose infusion (intravenous).

Pathological.—
Increased.—
1. Maturity-onset diabetes mellitus.
2. Liver disease.
3. Acromegaly.
4. Cushing's syndrome.—
   a. Spontaneous.
   b. Steroid-induced.
5. Dystrophia myotonica.
6. Insulinoma.
7. Familial fructose and galactose intolerance.

LEVELS FOLLOWING GLUCOSE INGESTION (GLUCOSE-TOLERANCE TEST).—
Physiological.—Maximal serum insulin levels are reached at 30–60 minutes. Fasting levels are reached once more by 2–4 hours. The peak value reached varies greatly between individuals, and from day to day in a given individual.

Increased peak values are found in normal pregnancy and in some cases of simple obesity.

Pathological.—
Increased.—
1. A few diabetics.
2. Acromegaly.
3. Cushing's syndrome.
4. Liver damage.
5. Werner's syndrome.
6. Lipo-atrophic dystrophy.

Decreased.—
1. Flat insulin response is more characteristic of young ketotic diabetics who require insulin therapy. The insulin response is inversely proportional to the degree of glucose intolerance. Obese patients tend to have higher insulin response.
2. Hypopituitarism.
3. Hypo-adrenalism.

LEVELS FOLLOWING INTRAVENOUS GLUCOSE INJECTION.—

Physiological.—There is normally an almost immediate and rapid rise in serum insulin levels.

Pathological.—Excessive rises occur in acromegaly and liver disease. In clinical diabetes there may be delay in response and suppression of release of insulin.

LEVELS AFTER 1 g. TOLBUTAMIDE INTRAVENOUSLY.—

Serum insulin levels rise excessively in 5–10 minutes in cases of insulinoma.

LEVELS AFTER 1 mg. GLUCAGON INTRAVENOUSLY.—

Similar but less consistent rises in serum insulin occur in cases of insulinoma.

LEVELS AFTER ORAL L-LEUCINE 150 mg./kg. BODY-WEIGHT.—

Similar but even less consistent rises in serum insulin occur in cases of insulinoma.

REFERENCES.—Hales, C. N., and Randle, P. J. (1963), *Biochem. J.*, **88**, 137; McKiddie, M. T., and Buchanan, K. D. (1969), *Quart. J. Med.*, **38**, 445; Henderson, J. R. (1970), *Lancet*, **2**, 545.

INSULIN TEST MEAL (GASTRIC SECRETION RESPONSE TO INSULIN-INDUCED HYPOGLYCÆMIA).—

Induced hypoglycæmia causes vagal stimulation centrally and this results in gastric secretion.

After an overnight fast 15 units of soluble insulin are injected intravenously. Gastric samples are aspirated every 15 minutes for 2 hours.

Normal Result.—Free hydrochloric acid increases to a maximum titration value of 90 ml. $N/10$ NaOH.

Postvagotomy Result.—If the vagotomy (usually for peptic ulcer relief) has been successful, there is complete achlorhydria.

N.B.—**The test is only significant if achlorhydria persists after the blood-sugar level has fallen below 50 mg./100 ml.**

REFERENCE.—Brooke, B. N. (1949), *Lancet*, **2**, 1167.

INSULIN TOLERANCE TEST (BLOOD-GLUCOSE RESPONSE TO INSULIN-INDUCED HYPOGLYCÆMIA).—

After the patient has been on a full carbohydrate-rich diet for 3–7 days and has fasted on the morning of the test, blood is taken for fasting sugar estimation; 0·1 unit soluble insulin/kg. body-weight is injected intravenously and blood samples are collected at 5, 10, 15, 20, 30, 45, 60, 90, and 120 minutes. This is more frequent than is usually suggested, but in this way the maximum fall which can occur in the early stages is not missed.

Normal.—Rapid fall from a normal fasting level occurs, falling to as low as 30–40 mg./100 ml. (i.e., 50 per cent of the fasting level). This fall occurs before the first 20–30 minutes of the test. Subsequently the blood-sugar level rises to the fasting level within 90–120 minutes.

Pathological.—

1. *Decreased Tolerance.—*
   a. *Increased Insulin Sensitivity.*—An excessive fall in the blood-sugar may occur in:—
      i. Hyperinsulinism.—
         α. Due to pancreatic islet cell hyperplasia.
         β. Due to pancreatic islet cell adenoma.
         γ. Due to pancreatic islet cell carcinoma.

  ii. Adrenal cortical insufficiency.
 iii. Hypopituitarism with secondary adrenal in-
      sufficiency.
  iv. Hypopituitarism with secondary hypothyroidism.
   v. Some cases of von Gierke's liver glycogen storage
      disease.
  vi. Starvation prior to the test with liver glycogen
      depletion.
  b. *Hypoglycæmic Unresponsiveness.*—After the blood-
     sugar level has fallen it fails to rise again, i.e., there is
     little or no glycogenolysis in response to the low blood-
     sugar level. All the cases listed in (*a*) show this, and this
     is probably the more significant part of the test, i.e.,
     control blood-sugar level should normally be regained
     within 90–120 minutes.

N.B.—Glucose solution both for oral and intravenous
administration must be available during the test, as dangerous
coma may be precipitated in adrenal insufficiency and hypopituitarism. A smaller dose of insulin (0·03 unit/kg. body-
weight) should be given in suspected hypopituitarism.

  2. *Increased Tolerance.*—The blood-sugar falls by less than
     25 per cent of its initial value (i.e., not below 60 mg./100
     ml.) and rapidly returns to the fasting level:—
     a. Cushing's syndrome.
     b. Acromegaly.
     c. Some cases of diabetes mellitus, particularly the older,
        more adipose, patients.
     d. Thyroid deficiency and myxœdema.

  REFERENCE.—Fraser, R., Albright, F., and Smith, P. H. (1941), *J.
  clin. Endocrin.*, 1, 297.

INSULIN-TOLERANCE TEST.—Plasma cortisol secretion
response to insulin-induced hypoglycæmia.

Physiological.—Following insulin-induced hypoglycæmia, the
plasma cortisol level rises by more than 5–7 μg./100 ml. and
the maximal values exceeding 25 μg./100 ml. are attained within
90 minutes after the insulin injection.

Pathological.—
  Impaired or Absent Response.—
  1. Cushing's syndrome.
  2. Depressive illness. The response is less than normal,
     with increased response on recovery.
  3. Pathological change in the hypothalamic–pituitary
     axis. This test is more sensitive of minor change than
     the lysine vasopressin test, pyrogen test, or metyrapone
     test.
  4. Hypopituitarism. The test can be used to detect residual
     pituitary function following hypophysectomy, while the
     patient is still on replacement therapy with small doses
     of steroids.
  5. Adrenal failure. The damaged adrenals may be
     incapable of secreting cortisol.

REFERENCES.—Greenwood, F. C., Landon, J., and Stamp, T. C. B.
(1966), *J. clin. Invest.*, 45, 429; James, V. H. T., Landon, J., Wynn,
V., and Greenwood, F. C. (1968), *J. Endocrinol.*, 40, 15; Carroll, B. J.
(1969), *Brit. med. J.*, 3, 27; Jacobs, H. S., and Nabarro, J. D. N.
(1969), *Quart. J. Med.*, 38, 475.

(For growth hormone response to insulin-induced hypo-glycæmia, *see* GROWTH HORMONE IN PLASMA.)

INSULIN-GLUCOSE TOLERANCE TEST.—The procedure is as for the insulin tolerance test, but 0·8 g. glucose per kg. body-weight is given in water orally at the same time as the insulin is injected. This test can be used to differentiate between insulin-sensitive and insulin-resistant diabetes mellitus:—

1. *Insulin Sensitive.*—These patients show little change in blood-sugar level.
2. *Insulin Resistant.*—The blood-sugar level rises as in an ordinary glucose tolerance curve.

REFERENCE.—Himsworth, H. P. (1939), *Lancet*, **2**, 1, 65, 118, 171.

IODINE

PROTEIN-BOUND IODINE IN SERUM.—
Normal Range.—3·5–7·0 µg./100 ml. The serum protein-bound iodine is a measure of the circulating thyroxine. The serum level in the normal newborn infant is above normal for a few days.

Increase.—
1. Iodine therapy.—
   a. As inorganic iodine (acts for days–weeks).
   b. As organic compounds (acts for months).
   c. As antiseptic, when blood samples may be contaminated.
2. Œstrogen therapy.
3. In normal pregnancy the level may rise to 15 µg./100 ml. The level falls in threatened abortion.
4. Thyrotoxicosis. The blood level may range from 7 to 20 µg./100 ml. With treatment, the level falls to normal more rapidly than does the basal metabolic rate.
5. Acute hepatitis.

Decrease.—
1. Hypothyroidism. The serum level ranges from 0 to 3 µg./100 ml. After treatment with thyroid the level returns to normal in about 3 weeks.
2. Tri-iodothyronine therapy.
3. Malnutrition.
4. Nephrosis (the iodine-carrying alpha-globulin may be lost in the urine).
5. Cortisone therapy.
6. Thiocyanate therapy. Also chlorates, para-amino-salicylic acid, para-aminobenzoate, thiouracils, mercurial diuretics, all reduce the protein-bound iodine.
7. Cirrhosis of the liver.
8. Accidental hypothermia.

TRI-IODOTHYRONINE (T_3) UPTAKE TEST (*IN VITRO*).—
Serum from a patient is incubated with ^{131}I-tri-iodothyronine (^{131}I-T_3), the unbound ^{131}I-T_3 is removed by dialysis and ultra-filtration and the ^{131}I-T_3 binding power of the serum is determined. (Patient's red cells can also be used for the test.)

Increase.—Hyperthyroidism.
Decrease.—Hypothyroidism. Normal pregnancy.

REFERENCE.—Garnett, E. S., Pollard, A. C., and Webber, C. E. (1969), *Lancet*, **2**, 318.

URINE EXCRETION OF RADIOACTIVE IODINE.—The thyroid gland and the kidneys compete for circulating iodine.

Increased Urine Excretion.—
1. *Hypothyroidism.*—70–92 per cent of the dose is excreted in the urine in 48 hours, i.e., there is an overlap with the normal range.
2. *After Mercurial Diuretics.*

Normal Urine Excretion.—
1. 30–70 per cent may be excreted in the first 24 hours.
2. 44–88 per cent is excreted in 48 hours.

Decreased Urine Excretion.—
1. *Thyrotoxicosis.*—
   a. Less than 20 per cent of the dose is excreted in 24 hours.
   b. 6–35 per cent is excreted in 48 hours.
2. *Renal Disease.*—The renal iodide clearance is reduced in renal disease.

RADIOACTIVE IODINE UPTAKE BY THYROID GLAND.—
Normal.—20–50 per cent of administered dose is taken up by the thyroid in 24 hours. The uptake by the gland is normal in anxiety states. ^{132}I has a half-life of 2·26 hours, giving a smaller radiation dose. It is therefore preferable in children and pregnant women. Pregnant women should not be given radioactive material if it can possibly be avoided. Iodine uptake is inversely proportional to the daily ingestion of iodide.

Increased Uptake.—
1. *Hyperthyroidism.*—
   More than 30 per cent in 6 hours ⎫ Various workers
   More than 40 per cent in 4 hours ⎬ have different
   More than 55 per cent in 24 hours ⎭ criteria.
2. Compensatory hyperactivity without thyrotoxicosis (endemic goitre) due to low iodide intake in diet.
3. Gigantism and acromegaly (if BMR is increased).

Decreased Uptake.—
1. Hypothyroidism.—10–20 per cent is suggestive, less than 10 per cent is diagnostic.
2. Therapy with desiccated thyroid.
3. Hypopituitarism.

False Results are obtained:—
1. After iodide medication. The effects last up to 2 months after the last dose.
2. After a bronchogram, etc. The effects of organic iodine last much longer than 2 months.
3. Thiouracil therapy.
4. Addison's disease.
5. Renal disease ⎫ Due to reduced renal
6. Congestive cardiac failure ⎬ iodide clearance.

Diagnosis of Thyrotoxicosis.—
1. The BMR is accurate in 66 per cent of cases.
2. Serum protein-bound iodine is accurate in 80 per cent of cases.
3. Radioactive iodine uptake by the thyroid gland is accurate in 95 per cent of cases.

N.B.—

Tri-iodothyronine (T_3) Suppression Test.—

By giving 1-tri-iodothyronine (100 μg. per day for 1 week), the thyroid uptake is inhibited in euthyroid cases. Gland uptake is unaffected in hyperthyroidism. *' no longer under pit. control.*

Thyrotrophic Hormone (TSH) Stimulation Test.—

Following the injection of 10 U.S.P. units of thyrotrophin on 2 days, in the presence of panhypopituitarism:—

a. In atrophy of the thyroid there is no increase in uptake over the control value.

b. Where thyroid tissue is present, then uptake is greater than in the control reading.

References.—Wayne, E. J. (1960), *Brit. med. J.*, **1**, 1, 78; Hobbs, J. R., Bayliss, R. I. S., and MacLagan, N. F. (1963), *Lancet*, **1**, 8.

IRON

IRON IN SERUM.—

Normal Range.—79–196 μg./100 ml.

$$\left(\frac{\mu g./litre}{55 \cdot 85} = \mu mol./litre. \right)$$

Serum iron exists in the ferric state and is attached to the serum beta-globulin siderophilin (2 atoms of iron per molecule of protein). The normal adult body contains about 4 g. of iron, of which 3 g. are present in the red blood-cells: thus specimens for analysis must be free from any hæmolysis for some methods. There is a normal diurnal variation, with higher levels present in the early morning. Sleep deprivation or stress results in the diurnal variation being lost and serum iron levels falling.

Physiological.—

1. *Normal Pregnancy.*—Progressive fall from mid-term onwards, with rising total iron binding capacity.

2. *Normal Infant.*—150–200 μg./100 ml. at birth, with low total iron binding capacity. Falling to below 100 μg./100 ml. within a few hours. Adult levels reached by 3–7 years. Diurnal variation develops by 1–3 years.

Pathological.—

Increase.—

1. *Excessive Iron Intake:*—

a. Excessive intravenous or intramuscular iron therapy.

b. Repeated blood transfusions. Each pint of citrated blood contains more than 0·2 g. of iron.

c. Hæmochromatosis. In this condition there is excessive absorption of iron from the alimentary tract.

d. Acute iron poisoning, e.g., ingestion of ferrous sulphate tablets by very young children. Serum iron level may exceed 1000 μg./100 ml. and, untreated, death may occur within 6 hours.

N.B.—There is no mechanism for the excretion of excess iron. Women regularly lose 10–40 mg. of iron at each menstrual period. Paradoxically, this loss may be greater in the presence of iron deficiency anæmia.

During pregnancy the fœtus obtains 800–900 mg. of iron from the maternal circulation.

2. *Increased Rate of Blood Destruction.*—As in hæmolytic anæmias.

3. *Liver Disease.*—In both acute hepatitis and in active portal cirrhosis the serum iron level is increased, presumably due to the liberation of stored iron from necrosing liver cells. Circulating ferritin has been identified.
4. *Nephritis.*
5. *Refractory Anæmia.*—Iron absorption is normal, but iron is not being used because hæmoglobin synthesis is slowed.
6. Oral contraceptives.
7. Primary inherited sex-linked sideroblastic anæmia.
8. Acute leukæmia.

N.B.—**Where the serum iron level is raised, the serum iron binding protein is increased.**

Decrease.—
1. *Iron-deficiency Anæmia.*
2. *Remission in Pernicious Anæmia* (i.e., rapid blood regeneration uses up available iron).
3. *Acute and Chronic Infection.*—A low serum iron level frequently develops within 24 hours of onset.
4. *Carcinoma.*—Normal quantities of storage iron and increased red blood-cell turnover.
5. *Nephrosis.*—Probably related to loss of specific iron binding serum globulin in the urine.
6. *ACTH or Adrenocortical Extract Therapy.*—The serum iron level falls, lowest level being reached after 8 hours.
7. Post-operative decrease (probably related to stress reaction).
8. *Kwashiorkor.*
9. Congenital atransferrinæmia.

REFERENCES.—Reissmann, K. R., and Dietrich, M. R. (1956), *J. clin. Invest.*, 35, 588; Trinder, P. (1956), *J. clin. Path.*, 9, 170.

IRON BINDING CAPACITY OF SERUM.—The total serum iron binding capacity is a measure of the serum concentration of transferrin, the specific iron-carrying protein. Transferrin is present in the serum at a concentration of 250 mg./100 ml. The mean total=148 mg./kg. body-weight, 11·8 mg./kg. body-weight being degraded each day, giving a half-life of 8·8 days. Serum TIBC falls soon after birth and subsequently rises to about 400 μg./100 ml. by 2 years. Adult levels are reached later. Direct measurement of transferrin is difficult, and only performed in research laboratories.

The serum iron binding capacity consists of:—
1. *Total Serum Iron Binding Capacity (TIBC).*—Normal adult range 306–429 μg. of iron/100 ml. serum.
2. *Serum Unsaturated Iron Binding Capacity (UIBC).*—Normally about 35 per cent of the serum transferrin is bound with iron, i.e., UIBC=TIBC minus serum iron.

Physiological.—
Infants.—TIBC falls after birth, subsequently rising to about 400 μg./100 ml. by 2 years.
Pregnancy.—In normal pregnancy, the TIBC rises to about 450 μg./100 ml., while the serum iron falls, i.e., high UIBC.

N.B.—When iron salts are injected intravenously, toxic symptoms develop as soon as the iron binding capacity is exceeded.

1. Raised Serum Iron Binding Capacity (Total):—

a. *With Raised Serum Iron Concentration* (i.e., the total transferrin concentration is increased, but the unsaturated iron binding capacity is reduced):—

   i. Liver damage. Acute hepatitis and active portal cirrhosis.

   ii. Increased blood destruction, e.g., hæmolytic anæmia.

   iii. Excessive iron intake:—

     α. Prolonged parenteral iron therapy.

     β. Repeated blood transfusions in refractory anæmia.

     γ. Hæmochromatosis.

     δ. High iron diet with low phosphate content, e.g., Bantus using iron cooking pots.

b. *With Low Serum Iron Concentration* (i.e., high UIBC):—

   i. Normal pregnancy.

   ii. Acute and chronic blood-loss. The available iron is used for blood regeneration.

   iii. Some cases of iron deficiency, clearance rate is below normal.

2. Low Serum Iron Binding Capacity (Total) (UIBC normal or low):—

a. Acute and chronic infections. The serum iron falls proportionally more than the transferrin content.

b. Pernicious anæmia in relapse.

c. Uræmia.

d. Carcinomatosis.

e. Nephrotic syndrome. Excessive loss of protein bound iron in the urine.

f. Kwashiorkor. Serum transferrin is markedly reduced.

g. Scurvy.

h. Hæmolytic anæmia.

i. Rheumatoid arthritis. Low TIBC rises with successful steroid therapy.

j. Congenital transferrinæmia.

REFERENCES.—Jordan, A. (1956), *J. clin. Path.*, Broadsheet No. 14, Assoc. Clin. Pathologists; Ramsay, W. N. M. (1958), *Advances in Clinical Chemistry* (Ed. Sobotka and Stewart), pp. 2–32. New York: Academic Press; Awai, M., and Brown, E. B. (1963), *J. Lab. clin. Med.*, **61**, 363.

IRON IN URINE.—Urine iron excretion after desferrioxamine.—

Normal.—Adult males.—800 μg. iron excreted in 24 hours.

Pathological.—

Increase.—Iron overload. More than 2200 μg. iron excreted in 24 hours.

Decrease.—Iron deficiency with depleted iron stores—less than 600 μg. iron/24 hr. After a small dose of oral iron, less than 150 μg. iron are excreted (evidence of ineffective erythropoiesis in iron deficiency).

ISO-CITRATE DEHYDROGENASE IN CEREBROSPINAL FLUID

Normal Range.—0·03–0·2 unit/ml.

Pathological.—

Increase.—

1. Cerebral tumours (primary or secondary).
2. Cerebrovascular accidents.
3. Meningitis.

REFERENCES.—Sterkel, R. L., Spencer, J. A., Wolfson, S. K., and Williams-Ashman, H. G. (1958), *J. Lab. clin. Med.*, **52**, 176; Dawkins, M. J. R., MacGregor, W. G., and McLean, A. E. M. (1959), *Lancet*, **2**, 827.

ISO-CITRATE DEHYDROGENASE IN SERUM

The NADP-dependent variety of this enzyme catalyses the reaction:—

$$\text{D-Iso-citrate} + \text{NADP} \rightleftharpoons \text{Oxalosuccinate} + \text{NADPH}_2$$
$$\text{(TPN)} \qquad \text{(TPNH}_2)$$
$$\alpha\text{-oxaloglutarate} + CO_2$$

The highest tissue concentration of the enzyme is in the liver. It also occurs in heart muscle, skeletal muscle, and red blood-cells and platelets. Therefore hæmolysed specimens must be avoided.

Normal Range.—$0\cdot8-4\cdot4$ μmoles $NADPH_2$ formed per minute per litre at $25°$ C. (Partially destroyed if stored in deep freeze.)

Physiological.—

Increase.—Normal newborn serum level is higher than maternal serum level, reaching normal adult levels by the end of the first year.

Pathological.—

Increase.—

1. Early hepatitis (infective or homologous serum variety). Serum levels return to normal in second and third weeks (as do transaminases).
2. Drug hepatitis.
3. Glandular fever (i.e., associated hepatitis).
4. Kwashiorkor.
5. Secondary carcinomatosis of liver (moderate increases).
6. Carcinoma of pancreas.
7. Placental infarct.
8. Pre-eclamptic toxæmia. Frequently increased serum level, indicating placental degeneration within previous 48 hours.
9. Myeloid leukæmia.
10. Megaloblastic anæmia (serum levels 5 times normal).
11. Cystathionine synthetase deficiency (homocystinuria).

Serum levels are normal in:—

1. Myocardial infarction (unless associated liver hypoxia present).
2. Normal pregnancy.
3. Extrahepatic biliary obstruction.

Iso-enzymes of Iso-citrate Dehydrogenase.—There are four different iso-enzymes, but as yet they have not been found clinically useful.

KETONES

KETONES IN BLOOD.—Normally the blood level is less than 3 mg./100 ml.

Physiological.—

Increase.—

1. Starvation.
2. Severe carbohydrate restriction, with adequate fat intake.

Pathological.—

Increase.—

1. Untreated diabetes mellitus (up to 300–400 mg./100 ml. or more).
2. Post-pancreatectomy.
3. Von Gierke's liver glycogen storage disease, especially after fasting.
4. Fever ⎫
5. Thyrotoxicosis ⎬ Carbohydrate requirement increased.
6. Persistent vomiting and other causes of severe alkalosis.
7. Growth hormone administration.
8. Acromegaly.
9. 11-oxysteroid administration.
10. Cushing's syndrome.
11. After moderate doses of insulin the blood ketones tend to disappear. After prolonged excessive insulin administration ketosis develops, due to shortage of circulating glucose.

KETONES IN BREATH.—

Normal.—Less than 1·8 μg./litre.

Pathological.—

Increase.—

1. Carbohydrate starvation.
2. Diabetes mellitus.
   a. With increased blood-glucose.
   b. After overnight fast with normal blood-glucose.
   c. Patients controlled on reducing diet.
   d. Hypoglycæmia, especially in the morning in patients controlled with insulin.

The breath acetone correlates with plasma β-hydroxybutyrate concentration, and can be estimated by gas chromatography.

REFERENCE.—Tassopoulos, C. N., Barnett, D., and Fraser, T. R. (1969), *Lancet*, **1**, 1282.

KETONES IN URINE.—

Normal.—Less than 50 mg./100 ml.

Physiological.—

Increase.—

1. Starvation.
2. Severe carbohydrate restriction, adequate fat intake.

N.B.—**In either of these circumstances, children are more liable to develop ketosis than adults.**

Pathological.—

Increase.—

1. Unbalanced diabetes mellitus (up to 10–50 g./litre).
2. Persistent vomiting.
3. Von Gierke's liver glycogen storage disease, especially after fasting.
4. Fever.
5. Thyrotoxicosis.

6. Prolonged excessive insulin administration with low liver glycogen stores.
7. Severe renal glycosuria:—
   a. Renal tubule glucose reabsorption defect.
   b. Depletion of liver glycogen store following persistent glycosuria.
8. Secondary drowning (i.e., death in 4 days after immersion).

The qualitative detection of the presence of ketone bodies in the urine is adequate in clinical practice.

N.B.—**In the presence of renal tubular dysfunction in some cases of diabetes mellitus, with raised blood ketone levels, no ketone bodies appear in the urine.**

REFERENCE.—Irvine, R. E., and Rowell, N. R. (1956), *Lancet*, **2**, 1025.

LACTIC ACID IN BLOOD

Normal Range.—
Fasting, at rest, arterial blood—0·4–0·8 mEq./litre.
Fasting, at rest, venous blood—0·45–1·30 mEq./litre.

$$\left(\frac{mg./litre}{90} = mmol./litre.\right)$$

(Use of a tourniquet prior to venepuncture increases the lactic acid concentration.)

Pathological.—

Increase.—
1. Lactate/pyruvate ratio normal.—
   a. Pyruvate infusion.
   b. Glucose infusion.
   c. Bicarbonate infusion.
   d. Glycogen storage disease, Type I.
2. Lactate/pyruvate ratio variable.—
   Hyperventilation.
3. Lactate/pyruvate ratio increased.—
   a. Exercise.
   b. Epinephrine.
   c. Shock.
   d. Cardiopulmonary bypass.
   e. Acute hypoxæmia.
   f. Severe anæmia.
   g. Leukæmia.
   h. Diabetes mellitus.
   i. Phenformin therapy.
   j. Alcohol ingestion.
   k. Idiopathic lactic acidosis (associated with neural damage, and mental retardation).

In glycogen storage disease Type V (phosphorylase deficiency) the normal rise in blood lactate after ischæmic exercise does not occur.

REFERENCES.—Marbach, E. P., and Weil, M. H. (1967), *Clin. Chem.*, **13**, 314; Oliva, P. B. (1970), *Amer. J. Med.*, **48**, 209; Sussman, K. E., Alfrey, A., Kirsch, W., Zweig, P., Felig, P., and Messner, F. (1970), *Ibid.*, **48**, 104.

LACTATE DEHYDROGENASE IN CEREBROSPINAL FLUID

Increase.—

1. Intracerebral meningeal deposits of carcinoma, leukæmia, or lymphosarcoma. Normal results in primary tumours of the central nervous system.
2. Acute meningitis.
3. Subarachnoid hæmorrhage.
4. Cerebrovascular accident.

LACTIC ACID DEHYDROGENASE IN SERUM

The enzyme catalyses the reaction:—

$$\text{Pyruvate} + \text{DPNH} + \text{H}^+ = \text{Lactate} + \text{DPN}^+$$

Normal Range.—200–680 units/ml. serum (50–200 i.u./litre). The enzyme is predominantly intracellular. Red blood-cells contain 100 times the normal serum level. Therefore, absence of hæmolysis during collection of a blood sample for analysis is essential.

Physiological.—

Increase.—During normal pregnancy.

In normal newborn. ? evidence of some anoxic damage, reaching normal adult levels by the sixth day.

Pathological.—

Increase.—

1. Myocardial infarction. The serum level rises 2–10-fold after the first 12 hours and reaches a peak by 24–48 hours. The increase in serum concentration is roughly parallel to the degree of cardiac damage and also to the serum glutamic-oxalacetic transaminase level (SGOT).
2. Acute hepatitis.
3. Muscle damage, e.g., surgery.
4. Disseminated secondary carcinoma deposits, especially if present in the liver.
5. Myeloid leukæmia (high enzyme content of neutrophils).
6. Erythroblastosis fœtalis ⎫
7. Hæmolytic anæmia, es- ⎬ Derived from red blood-cells.
pecially if intravascular ⎭

Following ball-valve heart prosthesis insertion, serum lactate dehydrogenase activity rises in inverse proportion to the red-cell life.

8. Progressive muscular atrophy, especially in the early stages.
9. Pneumonia.

Increase in some cases of:—

1. Acute pancreatitis.
2. Dermatomyositis.
3. Renal disease.
4. Megaloblastic anæmia. SLD activity and red-cell count inversely related in folic acid and/or vitamin-B_{12} deficiency.
5. Acute rheumatic carditis.
6. Progressive muscular dystrophy.
7. Pulmonary infarction (some cases).

The serum level is unchanged in:—
1. Pulmonary infarction (some cases).
2. Pericarditis.
3. Chronic lymphatic leukæmia.
4. Aleukæmic leukæmia.

REFERENCES.—Wroblewski, F., and La Due, J. S. (1955), *Proc. Soc. exp. Biol., N.Y.*, **90**, 210; Wroblewski, F. (1957), *Amer. J. med. Sci.*, **234**, 301; Blanchaer, M. C., Green, P. T., Maclean, J. P., and Hollenberg, M. J. (1958), *Blood*, **13**, 245; Strandjord, P. E., and Clayson, K. J. (1961), *J. Lab. clin. Med.*, **58**, 962; Editorial (1962), *Brit. med. J.*, **2**, 1669; Elliott, B. A., and Wilkinson, J. H. (1962), *Lancet*, **2**, 71; Myhre, E., and Rasmussen, K. (1970), *Ibid.*, **1**, 355.

Serous fluid bathing malignant tumours, e.g., pleural effusion or ascites, has raised enzyme content.

Alpha-Hydroxybutyrate Dehydrogenase in Serum (SHBD)

SLD iso-enzyme studies show that the enzyme from heart muscle is much more stable at 65° C. than that from other tissues. It has recently been found that while oxalate inhibits the iso-enzyme from cardiac muscle more than that from liver, urea inhibits the liver iso-enzyme more than that from cardiac muscle. It is possible to estimate the iso-enzyme from cardiac muscle by using alpha-oxobutyrate as substrate in place of pyruvate (the so-called "serum alpha-hydroxybutyrate dehydrogenase" or SHBD).

Normal Values.—53–144 i.u./litre.

Pathological.—
Increase.—
1. Myocardial infarction. The serum level is raised abnormally for a longer period than when lactate dehydrogenase is estimated, and the SLD/SHBD ratio, which is normally 1·18–1·60, falls to less than 1·18.
2. Hepatitis. The SHBD level is only minimally raised, and the SLD/SHBD ratio is increased to 1·60–2·0.
3. Muscular dystrophy (especially in children).
4. Folic acid and/or vitamin-B_{12} deficiency.
5. Accidental hypothermia.

REFERENCES.—Pagliaro, L., and Notarbatolo, A. (1962), *Lancet*, **1**, 1043; Wilkinson, J. H. (1962), *An Introduction to Diagnostic Enzymology*, p. 158. London: Edward Arnold; Elliott, B. A., and Fleming, A. F. (1965), *Brit. med. J.*, **1**, 626; Johnston, H. A., Wilkinson, J. H., Withycombe, Wendy A., and Raymond, S. (1966), *J. clin. Path.*, **19**, 250.

PLACENTAL LACTOGEN IN PLASMA

This protein, which is solely of trophoblastic origin, is detectable in the maternal plasma by the 5th week of pregnancy, reaches a plateau by the third trimester, and falls rapidly after delivery of the placenta. It is detectable by radioimmunoassay, and it has been suggested that plasma levels are related to the placental weight. The value of this estimation is not established yet. It may complement œstriol estimations (which measure the ability of the fœtal adrenals to produce 16-α-dehydroepi-androsterone and the ability of the placenta to convert this substance to œstriol).

Increased.—
1. Multiple pregnancy.
2. Some diabetics with large placentas.

Decreased.—
1. Retarded fœtal growth due to placental insufficiency.
2. Falling levels reflecting altered placental function.—
    a. Toxæmia.
    b. Diabetes mellitus.
    c. Rhesus immunization.
    d. Sickle-cell anæmia.
3. Fifty per cent fall in late pregnancy has been taken as an indication for prompt induction of labour or for Cæsarean section.
4. Low levels have been found a few days before spontaneous abortion.

REFERENCES.—Editorial (1969), *Brit. med. J.*, **3**, 668; Editorial (1969), *Lancet*, **2**, 1405; Genazzani, A. R., Aubert, M. L., Casoli, M., Fiore Hi, P., and Felber, J.-P. (1969), *Ibid.*, **2**, 1385.

LACTOSE TOLERANCE TEST

After an overnight fast, 1·5 g. lactose per kg. body-weight is given orally in 400 ml. of water. Blood-glucose samples are taken at 0, 15, 30, 45, 60, and 120 minutes afterwards.

Normal.—The blood-glucose level rises by more than + 25 mg./100 ml. at 15–30 minutes.

Pathological.—The blood-glucose fails to rise by 25 mg./100 ml. or more.

1. *Primary Alactasia.*—Flattened lactose tolerance curve, with diarrhœa and the presence of lactose and abnormal amounts of amino-acids in the urine, while the subject is eating lactose-containing foods.
2. *Secondary Acquired Disaccharidase Deficiency.*—
    a. Milk intolerance.
    b. Sprue syndrome.
    c. Transient lactose intolerance associated with acute gastro-enteritis.
    d. Post-gastrectomy.

It has been suggested that lactose intolerance in otherwise normal adults with alactasia results from prolonged elimination of milk and milk products from the diet.

REFERENCES.—Cuatrecasas, P., Lockwood, D. H., and Caldwell, J. R. (1965), *Lancet*, **1**, 14; Editorial (1965), *Brit. med. J.*, **2**, 128; Sheehy, T. W., and Anderson, P. R. (1965), *Lancet*, **2**, 1.

LÆVULOSE TOLERANCE TEST

Lævulose 45–50 g. in 200 ml. of water is given orally. Blood samples are collected, ½-hourly for 2 hours with fasting.

Results.—
1. Normal fasting blood lævulose—less than 8 mg./100 ml.
2. Normal peak during test—less than 15 mg./100 ml.
3. Normal 2-hour reading—0–10 mg./100 ml.
    (All blood levels estimated as lævulose.)

Pathological.—In hepatic damage the blood level may rise to 16–20 mg./100 ml. during the 2-hour period.

In glycogen storage disease Type I the blood glucose does not rise after oral lævulose.

N.B.—Ten per cent of normal individuals excrete lævulose in the urine during the test. The test can only be used as a crude index of severe liver damage.

REFERENCE.—Herbert, F. K., and Davison, G. (1938), *Quart. J. Med.*, N.S., **7**, 355.

LEAD

LEAD IN BLOOD.—
Normal Value.—Less than 80 μg./100 ml.

$$\left(\frac{\mu g./litre}{207} = \mu mol./litre. \right)$$

The blood lead may be increased in acute lead poisoning, but may be within the upper limits of normal in chronic lead poisoning. In children beware of unexplained encephalitis, raised intracranial pressure, obscure anæmia, renal glycosuria, and abdominal pain, as manifestations of lead poisoning. Lead is laid down in the bones; thus, should metabolic acidosis develop, lead is liberated with calcium and the blood-lead level rises.

Blood-lead levels of more than 100 μg./100 ml. indicate lead poisoning. Following treatment with a chelating agent (calcium disodium ethylenediamine-tetra-acetate) the blood level falls to low normal values.

REFERENCES.—Brown, A. (1946), *Quart. J. Med.*, **15**, 77; Cotter, L. H. (1953), *J. Amer. med. Ass.*, **155**, 906; Leckie, W. J. H., and Tompsett, S. L. (1958), *Quart. J. Med.*, **27**, 65; Editorial (1959), *Lancet*, **1**, 1189.

LEAD IN URINE.—
Normal Output.—Less than 80 μg./24 hr.
Increased Output.—In lead poisoning the urine output of lead may increase to more than 100 μg./24 hr. This may be associated with an increased output of urine coproporphyrin III.

In chronic lead poisoning the blood-lead level may be within normal limits (i.e., less than 80 μg./100 ml.) and the urine excretion may be at the upper limit of normal. After the administration of the sodium-calcium salt of ethylenediamine-tetra-acetic acid, up to 2000 μg. of lead may be safely excreted in the urine in 24 hours. Thus the diagnosis becomes obvious, and also successful treatment has been initiated.

REFERENCES.—Kehoe, R. A., Thamann, F., and Cholak, J. (1935), *J. Amer. med. Ass.*, **104**, 90; Bradley, J. E., and Powell, A. M. (1954), *J. Pediat.*, **45**, 297.

LEUCINE AMINOPEPTIDASE IN SERUM

Aminopeptidases split amino-acids with a free amino group from amino-acid chains in peptides. Leucine aminopeptidase is estimated by its action on synthetic substrates.

The highest concentration of the enzyme is in the pancreas and liver.

Normal Range.—4·5–19·3 units/ml.
Pathological.—
Increase.—
1. Carcinoma of pancreas (variable serum levels) especially if there is no associated increase in either serum alkalin

phosphatase or serum aspartate aminotransferase (SGOT).

2. **Liver disease (hepatitis, cirrhosis).** Serum levels moderately increased.

3. **Cholecystitis.** Moderate increase.

4. **Pancreatitis.** Transient moderate rise in acute pancreatitis but no increase in serum levels in chronic pancreatitis.

5. **Secondary carcinomatous invasion of liver.** Moderate increase in serum level, which occurs even in the absence of jaundice (especially if steroids given).

6. **Simple bile-duct obstruction.** Variable increase in serum levels.

7. **Diffuse skin mastocytosis** (especially after skin friction).

8. **Pregnancy.** High serum levels are found prior to abortion.

9. **Nephrosis.**

10. **Some skin diseases.**

This test offers no special advantage over serum alkaline phosphatase. It may be used to detect secondary carcinoma in liver in cases in which the pancreas is not the primary site.

REFERENCES.—Harkness, J., Roper, B. W., Durant, J. A., and Miller, H. (1960), *Brit. med. J.*, **1**, 1787; Pruzanski, W. (1966), *Amer. J. med. Sci.*, **251**, 685.

LEUCINE AMINOPEPTIDASE IN URINE

Pathological.—

Increase.—

1. **Carcinoma of pancreas.** Marked increase.

2. **Simple bile-duct obstruction.** Moderate increase.

Not a useful test.

LEUCINE SENSITIVITY TEST

After an overnight fast an initial fasting blood-glucose sample is taken. A suspension of L-leucine (150 mg. per kg. body-weight) in water is given by mouth. Blood samples are then collected every 15 minutes for 1 hour.

Normal Result.—Slight fall in blood-glucose level only (5–15 mg./100 ml.).

Abnormal Result.—Blood-glucose level falls 40 per cent or more of initial blood-glucose level, usually within the first 30 minutes:—

1. **Idiopathic hypoglycæmia of children**; with leucine sensitivity.

2. **Patients being treated with sulphonylureas.**

3. **Insulinoma.**

REFERENCE.—Marks, V., and Rose, F. C. (1965), *Hypoglycæmia*. Oxford: Blackwell.

LIPASE IN SERUM

Lipase estimation includes: ali-esterases; cholinesterases; sterol esterases; lipoprotein esterases (heparin-clearing factor); pancreatic lipase (hydrolyses long-chain fatty acids from glycerol).

Speed of lipolysis: triglyceride > 1,2-diglyceride > 1,3-diglyceride > 1-monoglyceride.

Speed of reaction also affected by molecule size, and by degree of hydration of fatty acid, e.g., oleyl oleate is attacked slowly.

Thus the reaction is non-specific and the substrate used is critical.

Normal Range.—

1. 0–1·0 unit/ml.
2. 1·0–2·0 units/ml. is regarded as equivocal.
   (1 unit = titration of 1 ml. $N/20$ NaOH under the conditions of the test.)

Pathological.—

Increase.—

1. *Acute Pancreatitis.*—During the acute attack, the level may remain abnormally raised for 3 days (cf. rapid fall of blood amylase).

2. *Conditions involving the Pancreas.—*
   a. Carcinoma.
   b. Chronic biliary disease.
   c. Peptic ulcer perforating on to the pancreas

The advantage of the test is that the serum level subsides less rapidly than the serum amylase after an attack of acute pancreatitis. Also non-pancreatic conditions appear to have relatively less effect on the serum lipase than on the serum amylase.

REFERENCES.—Vogel, W. C., and Zieve, L. (1963), *Clin. Chem.*, **9**, 168 (improved method); Brockerhoff, H. (1968), *Biochim. biophys. Acta*, **159**, 296.

LIPIDS IN SERUM

Normal Range.—From 400 to 700 mg./100 ml.

The total serum lipids consist of:—

1. Neutral fats.
2. Phospholipids.
3. Cholesterol.

Physiological.—

1. In pre-adolescence the serum lipids are low.

2. In pregnancy the total serum lipids rise to a maximum by the 30th week, and regain pre-pregnancy levels by the 8th week post-partum. The increase is due to equal rises in cholesterol and phospholipids.

3. After a mixed meal containing plenty of fat the total serum lipids rise within 2 hours, reaching a maximum peak by 6–8 hours, and falling to the pre-prandial level by about 10 hours after the meal.

4. The relationship between lipids, lipoproteins, and atherosclerosis is not yet clear.

Pathological.—

Increase.—

1. *Increase in Cholesterol, Phospholipids, and Neutral Fats.—*
   a. *Essential Hyperlipœmia.*—The increase is mainly in neutral fats, and the serum is lactescent. The level of

total lipids may reach up to 8 g./100 ml., with serum cholesterol of more than 400 mg./100 ml. and phospholipids of more than 450 mg./100 ml. Either dairy fats or alcohol will cause a significant rise in the serum lipids in this condition.

REFERENCE.—Amatuzio, D. S., and Hay, L. J. (1958), *Arch. intern. Med.*, **102**, 173.

    b. Diabetes Mellitus.—In ketosis free fatty acids are also increased due to excessive fat mobilization and incomplete fat catabolism.

    c. Nephrosis.—The increase in neutral fat is only moderate. The major increase occurs in phospholipids and cholesterol.

    d. Relapsing Chronic Pancreatitis.

    e. Von Gierke's Liver Glycogen Storage Disease.—Rarely there is an increase in the serum lipids, which is associated with impaired carbohydrate metabolism and associated ketosis.

    f. Acute Hepatitis.

    g. Many patients with proven fatty livers.

    h. Zieves's syndrome.

2. *Increase in Cholesterol and Phospholipids.*—
    a. Biliary cirrhosis.
    b. Hypothyroidism.
    c. Cholangiolitic cirrhosis.
    d. Xanthomatosis. Hereditary condition with markedly increased lipids, especially cholesterol. The fasting serum is clear.

3. *Increase in Phospholipids and Neutral Fats, with Falling Serum Cholesterol.*—
    a. Terminal cachexia.
    b. Terminal uræmia (presumably associated with a low food intake, and also tissue catabolism).

Decrease in all Three Fractions.—
1. Acute infections.
2. Severe hypochromic anæmia.
3. Severe pernicious anæmia, in relapse. The red cell phospholipid is also decreased.
4. Hyperthyroidism.
5. Post-hepatitis, especially if hepatitis is superimposed on pre-existing cirrhosis.

REFERENCE.—Kunkel, H. G., Ahrens, E. H., and Eisenmenger, W. J. (1948), *Gastroenterology*, **11**, 499.

TOTAL ESTERIFIED FATTY ACIDS (TEFA) IN SERUM

The serum total esterified fatty acids consist of:—
    Ester cholesterol,
    Triglycerides,
    Phospholipids.

Normal Values.—450–750 mg./100 ml.
    Fasting—less than 500 mg./100 ml.
    Fatty meal—peak values at 6 hours, falling to initial levels by 24 hours.

Pathological.—

Raised.—

1. Hypercholesterolæmia.
2. Hyperlipæmia.

Following the introduction of clofibrate (ethyl ester of chlorophenoxyisobutyric acid) estimation of TEFA is preferred to estimation of serum cholesterol alone, especially in cases apparently liable to coronary artery thrombosis. Reduction in the serum cholesterol, triglycerides, and phospholipids can be followed during treatment with clofibrate.

REFERENCES.—Schon, H., and Zellar, W. (1962), *Münch. med. Wschr.*, **104**, 2433; Freedman, M. J., Frajola, W. T. (1963), *Amer. J. med. Sci.*, **246**, 277; Best, M. M., and Duncan, C. H. (1966), *Arch. intern. Med.*, **118**, 97; Lane, R. F. (1966), personal communication.

LIPIODOL TEST

No dietary restriction is required, apart from cessation of any pancreatic enzyme therapy for at least 48 hours.

Lipiodol 0·5 ml./kg. body-weight is given orally to children weighing 10–20 kg. (not less than 5 ml. or more than 10 ml. is given).

Urine is collected at 12, 18, and 24 hours for iodide estimation. It is suggested that pancreatic lipase splits the lipiodol, the liberated iodine being absorbed and subsequently excreted in the urine.

Results.—Iodine is normally detectable in a 1 : 8 dilution of urine, and usually in a 1 : 32 dilution.

In fibrocystic disease of the pancreas, iodine may only be detected faintly in a 1 : 1 dilution of urine.

*N.B.—***In severe illness in the absence of fibrocystic disease, the iodine excretion may be grossly reduced.**

French workers have used this test in adults in an attempt to detect chronic pancreatitis.

REFERENCE.—Silverman, F. N., and Shirkey, H. C. (1955), *Pediatrics*, **15**, 143.

NON-ESTERIFIED (FREE) FATTY ACIDS (NEFA) IN PLASMA

In the post-absorptive state 50–90 per cent of the body energy requirements are met by circulating free fatty acids in the plasma. Normally up to 25 g. of fatty acids are transported per hour in the body in this way, which means that the estimation of NEFA in plasma at random is not very useful clinically. In any case, it is important that chilled heparinized plasma is used for the estimation.

Normal Range.—0·45–0·9 mEq./litre.

Physiological.—

*Increase.—*Starvation.

*Decrease.—*Food.

Pathological.—

Increase.—

1. Diabetic ketosis.
2. Post-myocardial infarction, especially with serious arrhythmias.

3. Stress (mobilization of NEFA after stress is apparently less in asthmatics than in controls. ? Evidence of decreased adrenal medullary activity).

REFERENCES.—Henry, R. J. (1964), *Clinical Chemistry. Principles and Technics*, p. 871. Hoeber Medical Division. New York: Harper & Row; Fairweather, D. V. I., and Layton, R. (1967), *J. clin. Path.*, **20**, 665; Oliver, M. F., Kurien, V. A., and Greenwood, T. W. (1968), *Lancet*, **1**, 710; Mathe, A. A., and Knapp, P. H. (1969), *New Engl. J. Med.*, **281**, 234.

FAT IN URINE (LIPURIA).—

Normal.—Less than 25 mg./litre.
Pathological.—Lipuria has been described in:—
1. Nephrosis (some cases).
2. Diabetes mellitus, if unbalanced.
3. Chyluria.
4. Rarely after excessive fat intake, e.g., cod-liver oil.
5. After fracture of a long bone, i.e., yellow marrow is released.
6. After severe crush injury.
7. Phosphorus poisoning.
8. Severe alcohol poisoning.

REFERENCE.—Broder, G. (1969), *Lancet*, **2**, 188.

LITHIUM IN SERUM

Lithium salts have been found to be useful in the treatment of psychotic excitement in manic-depressive patients. The optimum serum concentration appears to be 0·5–1·5 mEq./litre (mmol./litre). Above this concentration signs of toxicity occur when the serum concentration exceeds 2·0 mEq./litre. Serum concentrations of less than 0·5 mEq./litre are ineffective.

Toxicity may develop even when serum concentrations are within the therapeutic range, and this may be related to raised lithium levels in the cerebrospinal fluid. This was suggested by the finding of serum levels exceeding 11 mEq./litre with cerebrospinal fluid levels of less than 1 mEq./litre in a case of acute suicidal attempt. No toxic symptoms or signs occurred in this case, suggesting active transfer mechanisms involved in moving lithium from the blood to the cerebrospinal fluid.

Lithium appears to cause a decrease in cerebral glutamate (which is thought to be an excitatory transmitter). It also reduces production of cyclic-adenosine monophosphate, particularly in the brain.

Increased excretion of lithium in urine occurs following intravenous sodium bicarbonate, sodium lactate, or amino-phylline. Oral sodium chloride supplements may reduce the incidence of lithium toxicity. In the kidney 70 per cent reabsorption occurs.

REFERENCES.—Schou, M. (1968), *J. Psychiat. Res.*, **6**, 67; Thomsen, K. (1969), *Acta psychiat. scand.*, Suppl. 207, 83; Bleiweiss, H. (1970), *Lancet*, **1**, 416; Dousa, T., and Hechter, O. (1970), *Ibid.*, **1**, 834; De Feudis, F. U., and Delgado, J. M. R. (1970), *Nature, Lond.*, **225**, 749; Coombs, H. I. (1971), *Brit. J. Psychiat.*, in press.

LYSINE VASOPRESSIN TEST OF HYPOTHALAMIC-PITUITARY–ADRENAL FUNCTION

After injection of lysine vasopressin plasma cortisol concentrations increase in normal subjects by more than 6 μg./100 ml. Growth-hormone response is variable and no consistent results have been obtained in normal subjects. The response to insulin-induced hypoglycæmia is probably a more sensitive test of minor changes in the hypothalamic–pituitary–adrenal axis.

REFERENCES.—Greenwood, F. C., and Landon, J. (1966), *J. clin. Path.*, **19**, 284; Carroll, B. J., Pearson, Margaret J., and Martin, F. R. (1969), *Metabolism*, **18**, 476; Jacobs, H. S., and Nabarro, J. D. N. (1969), *Quart. J. Med.*, **38**, 475.

MAGNESIUM

MAGNESIUM IN SERUM.—

Normal Range.—1·8–3·6 mg./100 ml. (1·5–3·0 mEq./litre).

At least 70–85 per cent is in a diffusible state; 35 per cent of serum magnesium is protein-bound.

$$\left(\frac{\text{mg./litre}}{24\cdot3} = \text{mmol./litre.}\right)$$

At least 70–85 per cent is in a diffusible state.

Pathological.—

Increase.—
1. Renal failure.
2. Liver disease.
3. Parenteral magnesium salts, with associated fall in serum calcium.
4. After glucose ingestion.
   The serum magnesium increases by about 0·6–0·8 mg./100 ml.
5. Oxalic acid poisoning, with an associated fall in serum calcium.

Decrease.—
1. Prolonged magnesium deprivation, e.g., prolonged intravenous maintenance therapy as in severe burns.
2. Renal disease with high urine output, for example in nephrosis.
3. Possibly in some cases of rickets.
4. Possibly during pregnancy in some cases.
5. Primary hyperaldosteronism.
6. Following parathyroidectomy in primary hyperparathyroidism.
7. Acute alcoholism.
8. Intestinal malabsorption.
9. Recessive sex-linked condition, with secondary hypocalcæmia, affecting boys.

There appears to be no definite clear-cut clinical syndrome of magnesium excess or deficiency. Excess may be associated with central nervous system and cardiac depression. Deficiency may be associated with neuromuscular irritability and tetany.

The serum magnesium/calcium ratio is normally 0·3 ± 0·06, range 0·22–0·50, and the ratio tends to rise in both renal and pulmonary disease, and fall following biliary obstruction.

REFERENCES.—Smith, A. J. (1955), *Biochem. J.*, **60**, 522; Hanna, S., North, K. A. K., MacIntyre, I., and Fraser, R. (1961), *Brit. med. J.*, **2**, 1253; Vainsel, M., Vandevelde, G., Smulders, J., Vosters, M., Hubain, P., and Loeb, H. (1970), *Arch. dis. Childh.*, **45**, 254.

MAGNESIUM IN URINE.—
Normal Output.—0·172–0·285 g./24 hr.
Of the total daily output (which equals the intake in the diet):—

1. 20–50 per cent appears in the urine.
2. 80–50 per cent appears in the fæces.

N.B.—It appears that in some patients who repeatedly form renal stones, the urine magnesium output is reduced, and the magnesium/calcium ratio is lower than in controls.

REFERENCE.—Oreopoulos, D. G., Soyannwo, M. A. O., and McGeown, M. G. (1968), *Lancet*, 2, 420.

MALATE DEHYDROGENASE IN SERUM

The enzyme catalyses the reaction:—

$$\text{L-Malate} + \text{NAD} \rightleftharpoons \text{oxaloacetate} + \text{NADH}_2$$
$$\text{(DPN)} \qquad\qquad\qquad \text{(DPNH}_2\text{)}$$

The highest tissue concentrations are found in heart muscle, skeletal muscle, liver, and kidney. Red cells also contain a high concentration of the enzyme, and therefore hæmolysis of specimens must be avoided.

Normal Range.—50–104 units.

Normal newborn infant. Raised serum levels are found, which may be evidence of anoxia and tissue damage during birth.

Pathological.—

Increase.—

1. Active intravascular hæmolysis.
2. Myocardial infarction. Serum level rises after 6–24 hours to a peak at 24–48 hours (2–15 × normal), falling to normal by 5 days. The peak precedes SGOT and LDH, and degree is similar to rise in SGOT.
3. Hepatitis. Serum level rises in infective hepatitis, homologous serum jaundice, and also experimental toxic hepatitis.
4. Cirrhosis. Slight increase.
5. Pancreatitis. Slight increase.
6. Bile-duct disease. Slight increase.
7. Megaloblastic anæmia. Serum levels rise to up to 400 × normal value.

Study of iso-enzymes not yet of clinical use.

Results obtained with this enzyme are very similar to those obtained with serum lactate dehydrogenase.

REFERENCE.—Bing, R. J., Castellanos, A., and Siegel, A. (1957), *J. Amer. med. Ass.*, 164, 647.

MELANURIA

Melanin is a pigment derived from tyrosine, which is normally present in hair, skin, and various parts of the eye.

Pathological.—Melanin is normally absent from the urine. It appears in some cases of melanotic tumour, especially if there are secondary tumour deposits in the liver.

The freshly passed urine contains the colourless precursor melanogen, which is oxidized to black melanin on standing in air.

In patients with a confirmed diagnosis of malignant melanoma melanogenuria is associated with a poor prognosis. Melanogen excretion is reduced when cytotoxic drugs cause clinical improvement.

REFERENCE.—Crawhall, J. C., Hayward, B. J., and Lewis, C. A. (1966), *Brit. med. J.*, **1**, 1455.

MERCURIC CHLORIDE TURBIDITY TEST OF SERUM
(Takata-Ara Reaction)

Normal Range.—0 – +. Serum turbidity produced by a mercuric chloride solution is potentiated by gamma-globulin and by hepatitis beta-globulin, but is inhibited by normal albumin.

Increases in Turbidity.—
1. Cirrhosis of the liver.
2. Hepatitis.
3. Myeloma. (Gamma type.)
4. Sarcoidosis.
5. Pneumonia.
6. Tuberculosis.

N.B.—This test is not as sensitive as other empirical liver function tests. A recent modification has been developed in which the reagent is precipitated with beta- and gamma-globulin. While large amounts of albumin inhibit the reaction, small amounts actually enhance turbidity. This new modification is closely correlated with the zinc sulphate turbidity reaction, and less closely correlated with the thymol turbidity reaction and albumin/globulin ratio.

REFERENCE.—Maclagan, N. F., Bendandi, A., and Cooke, K. B. (1957), *Clin. chim. Acta*, **2**, 49.

MERCURY IN URINE

Normal Output.—Less than 100 μg./24 hr.

$$\left(\frac{\mu g./litre}{80} = \mu mol./litre. \right)$$

1. The estimation is occasionally of value where workers are exposed to mercury. Values of 2000 μg./24 hr. have been obtained in such cases.
2. In some infants with acrodynia (pink disease) values up to 200 μg./100 ml. have been recorded. The normal urine mercury output is up to 8 μg./100 ml.

REFERENCE.—Buckell, M. M., Hunter, D., Miller, R., and Perry, K. M. A. (1946), *Brit. J. industr. Med.*, **3**, 55.

METHÆMALBUMIN IN PLASMA

Methæmalbumin = Hæmatin linked with plasma albumin.
= Ferric compound of protoporphyrin linked with albumin.

Normally it is eliminated in the bile via the liver, in the form of coproporphyrin III.

Pathological Increase.—
1. Intravascular hæmolysis. The pigment is not normally detectable in the serum, but appears after rapid intravascular hæmolysis. During intravascular hæmolysis free

hæmoglobin is first bound by haptoglobins in the alpha-2 globulin fraction. As more hæmoglobin is liberated, it is taken up by the beta-1 globulin fraction. Finally when all the haptoglobin and beta-1 fraction are saturated, methæmalbumin is formed.

If there is associated liver damage with intravascular hæmolysis, the blood methæmalbumin level rises excessively, since excretion in the bile is reduced.

2. Acute hæmorrhagic pancreatitis. Methæmalbumin appears after 12 hours, reaching peak values by 4–5 days.

3. Small amounts of methæmalbumin may occur in some cases of Addisonian megaloblastic anæmia.

N.B.—Methæmalbumin does not appear in the serum in:—
1. Acholuric jaundice.
2. Sickle-cell anæmia.
3. Thalassæmia.

In these three conditions, hæmolysis is not intravascular.

REFERENCE.—Winstone, N. E. (1965), *Brit. J. Surg.*, **52**, 804.

METHÆMOGLOBIN IN BLOOD

Normal Concentration.—0·01–0·5 g./100 ml. of whole blood. Methæmoglobin is the oxidized form of hæm (i.e., the iron is in the ferric state), and has no respiratory function.

Methæmoglobin is normally present in the red blood-cells because it is constantly formed during glycolysis. There is also constant reconversion to hæmoglobin in normal red cells. Methæmoglobin remains in the red blood-cells unless hæmolysis occurs, when the pigment appears in the plasma and the urine. By causing a shift of the oxyhæmoglobin dissociation curve to the left (as does carbon monoxide), tissue anoxia may be caused by quite low concentrations.

Pathological.—
Increase.—
1. *Increased Rate of Formation.*—(Or possibly poisoning of the enzymes in red blood-cells responsible for rapid reconversion to hæmoglobin.)
   a. Acetanilid.
   b. Acetylsalicylic acid.
   c. Aniline (ingestion, or after contact with freshly dyed garments or marking ink).
   d. Antimony compounds.
   e. Antipyrine.
   f. Chlorates.
   g. Nitrites:—
      i. Excess in diet, or in drinking water.
      ii. Reduction by bacteria of nitrates to nitrites in the bowel.
      iii. Stored spinach grown in land over-fertilized with nitrates. Bacteria convert the excess nitrates to nitrite.
   h. Nitrobenzene.
   i. Pamaquin therapy.
   j. Permanganates.
   k. Phenacetin.

l. Phenazone.

m. Phenylhydrazine ⎫ The pigment may be present
n. Severe sepsis ⎬ free in the plasma.
o. Sulphonal. ⎭

p. Sulphonamides (sulphanilamide > sulphapyridine > sulphathiazole).

During hæmolytic crises the pigment may appear in the plasma.

2. *Decreased Rate of Conversion to Hæmoglobin.*—Congenital and idiopathic methæmoglobinæmia due to deficiency of co-enzyme Factor 1 (Gibson-Harrison Type).

3. *Rare Familial Type.*—This condition is inherited via a dominant gene. The abnormality is due to a fault in the formation of the prosthetic globin fraction of hæmoglobin. The hæmoglobin is abnormally easily oxidizable to methæmoglobin, and is hæmoglobin M.

N-METHYLNICOTINAMIDE IN URINE

Much of the excretion of nicotinic acid in the urine is in the form of *n*-methylnicotinamide (F_2).

Normal Output.—

1. 2–30 mg./24 hr. is excreted as free nicotinic acid.

2. 3–12·5 mg./24 hr. is excreted as *n*-methylnicotinamide.

Detection of *n*-methylnicotinamide in a urine specimen obtained before breakfast and after voiding the overnight urine excludes a nicotinic acid deficiency.

Various forms of "saturation test" have been suggested.

REFERENCE.—Huff, J. W., and Perlzweig, W. A. (1943), *J. biol. Chem.,* **150**, 395, 483.

METOPIRONE (MEPYRAPONE) TEST

Intravenous injection of metopirone (mepyrapone) causes interference with the intra-adrenal conversion of 11-deoxycortisol (compound S) to hydrocortisol and cortisol, by inhibiting the enzyme 11-beta-hydroxylase. This results in a fall in the plasma cortisol level, which stimulates ACTH secretion by the normal pituitary. (Hydrocortisol is a strong suppressant of ACTH secretion whereas 11-deoxycortisol is only a weak suppressant.) The increased secretion of ACTH results in a marked increase of adrenal cortical activity with a subsequent marked increase in the urinary output of 17-oxogenic (17-ketogenic) steroids.

N.B. This test should not be performed immediately after the ACTH stimulation test. It is also interfered with by exogenous steroids, opium alkaloids, and phenothiazine.

Normal Response.—

1. Urine 17-oxogenic steroid output on second day of test after intravenous metopirone = 30–110 mg./24 hr.

2. Plasma cortisol falls to half normal level by 90 minutes of intravenous injection of metopirone, rising to normal levels again by 4 hours (i.e., excessive secretion of ACTH overcomes metopirone inhibition of 11-beta-hydroxylase).

This normal response indicates an intact pituitary-ACTH-adrenal axis.

Pathological.—No increase in urine 17-oxogenic steroid output.—

1. Failure to produce block of enzyme activity.
2. Failure of pituitary to produce ACTH, i.e., hypopituitarism.
3. Unresponsive adrenal cortex. In this case the ACTH stimulation test is also abnormal.

Benign or malignant adrenal adenoma results in a negative test, whereas simple adrenal hyperplasia gives a greater than normal response with excessive output of 17-oxogenic steroids in the urine.

If the plasma cortisol levels are measured during the test, failure of the plasma cortisol level to rise after the initial fall at 90 minutes indicates:—

a. Hypopituitarism.
b. Autonomous adrenal tumour.

REFERENCES.—DiRaimondo, V. (1962), *Laboratory Tests in Diagnosis and Investigation of Endocrine Functions* (Ed. Escamilla, R. F.), p. 284. Philadelphia: F. A. Davis & Co.; Metcalf, Mary, G., and Beaven, D. W. (1968), *Amer. J. Med.*, 45, 176.

MUCOPOLYSACCHARIDE ACID IN URINE

Increased acid mucopolysaccharides are present in the urine in:—

Cases of gargoylism (Hurler's syndrome).

The screening tests devised to detect this substance are not sensitive enough to detect the slight increase in urine acid mucopolysaccharide excretion which occurs in:—

Disseminated lupus erythematosus.
Rheumatoid arthritis, etc.

REFERENCES.—Dorfman, A. (1958), *Pediatrics*, 22, 576; (1961), *Ibid.*, 27, 112; Denny, W., and Dutton, G. (1962), *Brit. med. J.*, 1, 1555.

MYOGLOBINURIA

Myoglobin is a ferrous-porphyrin complex with a molecular weight of 17,000 (hæmoglobin molecular weight = 68,000). Each molecule contains one atom of ferrous iron (hæmoglobin carries 4 atoms per molecule). On electrophoresis of serum containing myoglobin it does not travel with haptoglobin (cf. hæmoglobin).

In an adult 3 per cent of total muscle protein is in the form of myoglobin. Following muscle destruction the plasma myoglobin level is never high (cf. hæmolysis of red blood-cells and plasma hæmoglobin), probably because its relatively smaller molecule allows its rapid filtration by the kidneys. (Renal threshold about 15 mg./100 ml. serum.)

In an attack the urine contains the pigment, a number of pigmented casts, but usually very few red blood-cells (cf. hæmoglobinuria).

Pathological.—

1. *Sudden Muscle Damage.*—
   a. Ischæmia, e.g., thrombosis of an artery supplying a large muscle mass.
   b. Crush injury.
   c. High-voltage electric shock.

    d. Violent exercise and heat-stroke.
2. *Muscle Damage in Disease.*—Myoglobinuria is present in some cases resembling progressive muscular atrophy.
3. *Unidentified Toxic Substance.*—"Haff" disease. The unidentified poison occurred in fish caught in certain estuaries in North Germany and Sweden.
4. *Idiopathic.*—Some of the severe cases may be familial. Also, some cases are associated with severe renal damage during the attack.
5. *Paroxysmal Myoglobinuria in Horses.*—Myoglobinuria may occur in horses which have previously been on a high carbohydrate diet, after severe unaccustomed exercise. There is no equivalent human condition.
    In march hæmoglobinuria in man, the red blood-cells break down, the muscles being unaffected.
6. *McArdle's Syndrome.*—Transient attacks of myoglobinuria.
7. *Sea-snake bite.*—Myoglobinuria common after such bites.
8. Following eating of quail on certain Mediterranean islands, acute myalgia with myoglobinuria $1\frac{1}{2}$–9 hours later, increased by exercise.

REFERENCES.—Acheson, D., and McAlpine, D. (1953), *Lancet,* **2**, 372; Editorial (1964), *Ibid.,* **2**, 1166 (18 references); Vertel, R. M., and Knochel, J. P. (1967), *Amer. J. Med.,* **43**, 435; Ouzounellis, T. I. (1968) *Presse méd.,* **76**, 1863.

NITROGEN

NON-PROTEIN NITROGEN IN BLOOD.—
Normal Range.—18–30 mg./100 ml.

$$\left(\frac{\text{mg./litre}}{14} = \text{mmol./litre.}\right)$$

The blood non-protein nitrogen (NPN) consists of:—
1. Urea.
2. Uric acid.
3. Creatinine.
4. Amino-acids.
5. Ammonia.
6. Unknown substances.

Normal Partition.—
1. After a high protein diet, the blood NPN increases and 90 per cent is urea.
2. After a low protein diet, the blood NPN falls and 50 per cent or less is present as urea.
3. In late pregnancy, the blood NPN falls and the proportion due to urea is low.

Pathological.—
Increase (When the blood-urea increases):—
    1. *Pre-renal Azotæmia.—*
        a. Burns and shock (blood amino-acids are increased).
        b. Late cirrhosis. A normal or falling blood NPN with raised blood ammonia concentration is found in other cases.
    2. *Renal Azotæmia.*—As in acute and chronic nephritis. All fractions of NPN increase.
    3. *Post-renal Azotæmia.*—E.g., urinary tract obstruction. All fractions of NPN increase.

N.B.—In many conditions the blood NPN is normal, but the partition is abnormal. For example:—

1. *Eclampsia.*—Blood-urea tends to decrease, but amino-acids and "unknown substances" are increased.
2. *Myeloid Leukæmia.*—The blood NPN may be increased, and there is frequently a marked increase in blood uric acid.
3. *Myeloma.*—Similarly, there may be an increase in the fraction due to uric acid.

Decrease.—

1. Severe hepatic insufficiency.
2. Hepatic necrosis.

N.B.—**It is common practice in many laboratories to estimate the blood-urea concentration rather than the blood NPN, and to follow this by estimation of the other individual fractions (e.g., uric acid) as indicated clinically.**

NITROGEN IN FÆCES.—

Normal Output.—

1. 1–2 g./24 hr.
2. 0·5 g./24 hr. on a protein-free diet.

Increase.—

1. Severe diarrhœa.
2. Pancreatic disease, 3–9 g./24 hr., in:—
   a. Chronic pancreatitis.
   b. Pancreatic duct obstruction.
   c. Post-pancreatectomy.
3. Gastrocolic fistula.
4. Steatorrhœa, up to 3 g./24 hr., in:—
   a. Sprue.
   b. Idiopathic steatorrhœa.
   c. Cœliac disease.

REFERENCE.—Peters, J. P., and Van Slyke, D. D. (1932), *Quantitative Clinical Chemistry*, 2, 535. London : Baillière, Tindall & Cox.

NITROGEN BALANCE.—

Dietary Nitrogen.—10–15 g./24 hr.

Positive Balance (i.e., the body retains nitrogen, and intake exceeds output).—

1. Normal growth.
2. Pregnancy.
3. Growth hormone administration.
4. Androgens.
5. Physiological doses of thyroxine.
6. Acromegaly.
7. Recovery from a negative phase (e.g., convalescence)
8. Œstrogens and gonadotrophins have a weak action.

Negative Balance (i.e., the body loses nitrogen, and output exceeds intake).—

1. *Low Protein Diet.*
2. *Faulty Absorption.*—
   a. Pancreatic disease.
   b. Malabsorption syndromes.
   c. Excessive small intestine resection.

3. *Excessive Protein Breakdown.*—
   a. Thyroxine therapy in excess, also thyrotoxicosis.
   b. ACTH administration.
   c. Glucocorticoid administration.
   d. Cushing's syndrome.
   e. Diabetic ketosis.
   f. Wounds and infections (excess glucocorticoids released).
   g. Actual Excessive Loss of Protein.—
     i. Burns.
     ii. Nephrosis.
     iii. Excessive production of pus.
     iv. Hæmorrhage.

NITROGEN IN URINE.—

Normal Output.—10–15 g./24 hr.
1. The urine non-protein nitrogen consists on average of:—
   a. Urea—85 per cent (related to protein catabolism).
   b. Ammonium ions—3 per cent (related to body and urine pH).
   c. Creatinine—5 per cent (related to body muscle-mass).
   d. Uric acid—1 per cent (related to dietary purine).
   e. Amino-acids—traces < 2 per cent of total urine N (up to 500 mg./24 hr.).
   f. Unidentified residue—5 per cent.
2. The percentage of NPN which is urea is:—
   a. On high protein diet (120 g./24 hr.)—90 per cent.
   b. On low protein diet (6 g./24 hr.)—60 per cent.
   c. On carbohydrate and fat only—20 per cent.
   After any injury the urine nitrogen excretion increases.

   Urine Protein Nitrogen—*see* Protein in Urine.

5'-NUCLEOTIDASE IN SERUM

5'-Nucleotidase acts only on nucleotides phosphorylated on the fifth ribose carbon atom, e.g.,

   Adenosine-5'-phosphate$+H_2O \rightarrow$adenosine$+$phosphate.

Normal Range.—2–17 i.u./litre.
Pathological.—
  Increase.—
   1. Extra-hepatic biliary obstruction.
   2. Intra-hepatic biliary obstruction.
   3. Hepatitis (although low levels have been reported with very severe liver damage), especially if intra-hepatic cholestasis present.

Unlike serum alkaline phosphatase the serum 5'-nucleotidase level is not increased in relation to osteoblastic activity. No elevation is seen in serum levels in Paget's disease of the bone, osteomalacia, or secondary deposits of carcinoma in bone. Although this ability to distinguish between bone disease and other diseases not affecting the bones is useful clinically, in the author's laboratory no special advantage over the simple alkaline phosphatase estimation has been found in liver disease. On the contrary, it was found that 5'N estimations were inferior to alkaline phosphatase estimations in the differential diagnosis of liver disease.

REFERENCES.—Campbell, D. M. (1962), *Biochem. J.*, **82**, 34P; Davidge, R. C., and Philpot, G. R. (1966), *Proc. Ass. clin. Biochem.*, **4**, 38.

ŒSTROGENS IN URINE

Normal Ranges (μg./24 hr.).—

	Onset of Menstruation	Ovulation Peak	Luteal Maximum
Œstrone	4– 7	11–13	11–23
Œstradiol	0– 3	4–14	4–10
Œstriol	0–15	13–54	8–72

Pathological.—

Increase.—
1. Granulosa cell tumour ⎤
2. Luteoma of ovary ⎬ May be within normal range.
3. Thecoma of ovary ⎦
4. Liver disease.
5. Some testicular tumours.

Decrease.—
1. Primary ovarian failure.
2. Secondary ovarian failure.

GONADOTROPHIN STIMULATION TEST OF OVARIAN FUNCTION.—Following injection with pregnant mare's serum (PMS) gonadotrophin a rise in urine œstrone output with peak values on the seventh day (sixth to eighth) represents a response to gonadotrophin stimulation. After 18,000 i.u. of PMS.— Less than 15 μg./24 hr.=subnormal ovarian response; 15– 80 μg./24 hr.=normal ovarian response; more than 100 μg./ 24 hr.=ovarian hypersensitivity as with polycystic ovaries.

REFERENCE.—Swyer, G. I. M., Little, Valerie, Lawrence, Daphne, and Collins, J. (1968), *Brit. med. J.*, **1**, 349.

ŒSTROGENS IN CLOMIPHENE CITRATE-INDUCED OVULATION.—It has been found that clomiphene citrate will induce ovulation in otherwise anovulatory amenorrhœa. The drug can also be used to convert irregular and prolonged intervals between ovulation to more predictable regular ovulation. It will also induce ovulation in cases of irregular anovular menstruation associated with cystic glandular hyperplasia.

The presumptive sign of ovulation is the "ovulatory peak" of urine œstrogen excretion preceded by a rise in output of pituitary gonadotrophins, when fertilization can be arranged.

ŒSTRIOL IN URINE

The normal fœtal adrenals produce 16-alpha-dehydro-epiandrosterone which is metabolized in the normal placenta and excreted in the maternal urine as œstriol.

Pathological.—

*Increase.—*Fœtus affected by the virilizing form of congenital adrenal hyperplasia.

Decrease.—
1. Low birth-weight baby.
2. Pre-eclampsia.

3. Intra-uterine fœtal death.
4. Severe erythroblastosis.
5. Live anencephalic fœtus. The fœtal adrenal cortex is defective.
6. Following steroid therapy to the mother.

REFERENCES.—Oakey, R. E., Bradshaw, L. R. A., Eccles, S. S., Stitch, S. R., and Heys, R. F. (1967), *Clin. chim. Acta*, **15**, 35; Heys, R. F., Scott, J. S., Oakey, R. E., and Stitch, S. R. (1968), *Lancet*, **1**, 328.

OXALATE IN PLASMA

Normal Range.—0·06–0·3 mg./100 ml.

$$\left(\frac{mg./litre}{126} = mmol./litre. \right)$$

Pathological Increase.—Oxalate poisoning.

REFERENCE.—Zarembski, P. M., and Hodgkinson, A. (1967), *J. clin. Path.*, **20**, 283.

OXALATE IN URINE

Normal Output.—15–20 mg./24 hr.

Increased Output.—
1. Transient increase follows ingestion of certain fruits and vegetables, e.g., rhubarb, strawberries, spinach, tomatoes, sorrel, etc.
2. Primary hyperoxaluria, which causes nephrocalcinosis. Daily output = 100–400 mg. oxalic acid/24 hr.
   a. Primary hyperoxaluria with glycollic aciduria.
   b. Primary hyperoxaluria with L-glyceric aciduria.
3. Pyridoxine deficiency.
4. ? Variety of pyridoxine dependency.

Decreased Output.—Vitamin B$_6$ (pyridoxine) appears to reduce urine oxalate output (tryptophan increases urine oxalate output).

This may be useful in prevention of renal stone formation.

REFERENCES.—Archer, H. E., Dormer, A. E., Scowen, E. F., and Watts, R. W. E. (1958), *Brit. med. J.*, **1**, 175; Gershoff, S. N., and Prien, E. L. (1960), *Amer. J. Clin. Nutrition*, **8**, 812.

17-OXOSTEROIDS IN URINE
(17-KETOSTEROIDS)

NEUTRAL 17-OXOSTEROIDS IN URINE.—
Normal Output.—

Age	Male (mg./24 hr.)	Female (mg./24 hr.)
Birth	Very low	Very low
5 years	0·3– 4·0	Very low
10	0·5– 7·0	0·3– 5·0
20	3·0–20	2·0–15·0
30	4·0–26	3·0–20
40	4·0–24	2·0–15
50	2·0–16	1·5–11
>50	Falling	Falling

The total urine neutral oxosteroids consist of:—
1. Androgens, including metabolites of testosterone.
2. Adrenocortical androgens.
3. Oxosteroids derived from corticoids.

The main constituents of 17-oxosteroids are:—
1. Dehydroisoandrosterone.
2. Ætiocholanone.
3. Androsterone.

Since most of the urine 17-oxosteroids are derived from the adrenals, the estimation is not a useful measure of testicular function.

Administration of 17-methyl testosterone:—
1. It is not excreted as a 17-oxosteroid.
2. It decreases the output of 17-oxosteroids in the urine of patients in whom the only source could be adrenal, e.g., women, and male castrates.
3. It decreases the 17-oxosteroids derived from the testis, e.g., adrenal hyperplasia and Cushing's syndrome.

Pathological.—
Increased Output.—

1. *Pituitary.*—Cushing's syndrome (output may be normal).
2. *Sex Glands.—*
   a. *Male.—*
      i. Precocious puberty (high excretion for child's age).
      ii. Interstitial cell tumour of the testis.

N.B.—**Chorionepithelioma and other tumours of the testis have a normal to low excretion of 17-oxosteroids.**

      iii. Injection of testosterone. 50 per cent of the dose appears in the urine as 17-oxosteroids (cf. effect of methyl testosterone).
      iv. Injection of chorionic gonadotrophin. (The testis is stimulated.)

   b. *Female.—*
      i. The majority of ovarian tumours are associated with increased urine output of 17-oxosteroids. Where the tumour is an arrhenoblastoma the output is normal.
      ii. The upper limit of normal excretion is approached late in normal pregnancy.

3. *Adrenals.—*
   a. Adrenal hyperplasia.
   b. Adrenal adenoma.
   c. Adrenal carcinoma. The 17-oxogenic steroid output may be normal, and the output of dehydroisoandrosterone may be increased.
   d. Cushing's syndrome.
   e. Adrenogenital syndrome.
   f. Feminizing syndrome in males.
   g. Increase within normal limits follows major surgical operations.
   h. Administration of ACTH:—
      i. It causes a rise in output in both normals and in cases with adrenal hyperplasia.
      ii. In cases with adrenal adenoma or carcinoma, ACTH produces no increase.

    i. Administration of cortisone (50–100 mg. daily for 7 days) causes:—

       i. Decreased output in (*a*).

       ii. No change in output in (*b*) or (*c*).

N.B.—In (*g*) there is also an increase in **17-hydroxycorticoids.**

Decreased Output.—

1. *Pituitary.*—

    a. Hypopituitarism. Very low output.

    b. Pituitary tumour. Normal levels at first, falling to low levels as hypopituitarism develops.

    c. Pituitary infantilism.

2. *Sex Glands.*—In true hermaphroditism there is normal to low output.

    a. Males.—

       i. Gonadal agenesis. Normal to low output.

       ii. Gonadal dysgenesis.

       iii. Hypogonadal eunuchoidism. Low normal to low output.

       iv. Prepuberty testicular failure (cf. testicular failure at puberty, and testicular failure without signs of eunuchoidism; both have normal rates of excretion).

    b. Females.—

    Primary ovarian failure has no effect on the urine 17-oxosteroid excretion rate.

3. *Adrenals.*—

    a. Addison's disease.—

       i. Adult male: 1–4 mg./24 hr., mainly derived from the testis.

       ii. Adult female: 0–1 mg./24 hr.

    Since remnants of functioning adrenal gland nevertheless may be present in Addison's disease, the following rates of excretion may be found when clinical signs of Addison's disease are apparent:—

       i. Adult males: 3–7 mg./24 hr.

       ii. Adult females: 1–7 mg./24 hr.

    b. Administration of cortisone to a normal individual depresses the excretion of 17-oxosteroids in the urine.

4. *General Metabolic Disorders.*—

    a. Myxœdema and hypothyroidism.

    b. Hepatic disease.

    c. Chronic illness, starvation, and debility.

5. *Renal Disease.*—Output may be reduced in advanced disease.

REFERENCE.—Med. Res. Counc. Com. on Clinical Endocrinology (1951), *Lancet*, 2, 585.

17-OXOGENIC (KETOGENIC) STEROIDS IN URINE.—

The substances known as 17-oxogenic steroids are essentially derived from 17-hydroxycorticoids (which include cortisone and hydrocortisone and their metabolites).

Normal Output.—

Age	Male (mg./24 hr.)	Female (mg./24 hr.)
Birth	Up to 4·0	Up to 3·0
5 years	1·0– 5·0	1·0– 4·0
10	3·0–10·0	2·5– 8·0
20	5·0–25	4·0–15·0
30	6·0–26	5·0–17·0
>30	Falling	Falling

1. The normal 17-oxogenic steroid/neutral 17-oxosteroid ratio is more than 1·0.
2. After cortisone therapy, the urine 17-oxogenic steroid output increases in proportion to the dose.
3. After ACTH gel the urine 17-oxogenic steroid increases in normal individuals by 20–60 mg./24 hr. The maximum response in Addison's disease is + 3 mg./24 hr. Thus this is a much more sensitive index of adrenal function than the estimation of neutral 17-oxosteroids after ACTH.

Pathological.—
Increased Output.—
  1. Cushing's syndrome.
  2. Virilism.
  3. Precocious puberty of adrenal cortical origin.
Decreased Output.—
  1. Addison's disease
  2. Hypopituitarism.

Plasma cortisol estimation is far more sensitive a test than urine 17-oxogenic steroids, particularly in Cushing's syndrome.

REFERENCES.—Norymberski, J. K., Stubbs, R. D., and West, H. F. (1953), *Lancet*, **1**, 1276; Hubble, D. (1955), *Ibid.*, **1**, 1; Levell, M. J., Mitchell, F. L., Paine, C. G., and Jordan, A. (1957), *J. clin. Path.*, **10**, 72; Cope, C. L., and Black, E. G. (1959), *Brit. med. J.*, **2**, 1117; Cope, C. L. (1966), *Ibid.*, **2**, 847.

OXYGEN IN BLOOD

One g. of hæmoglobin when fully converted to oxyhæmoglobin will combine with 1·36 ml. of oxygen at NTP.

Thus, the *Oxygen Capacity* is a measure of the total effective hæmoglobin (oxyhæmoglobin and reduced hæmoglobin). Carboxyhæmoglobin, methæmoglobin, and sulphæmoglobin are not included. In Rhesus incompatibility due to 'blocking' antibodies, the oxygen-carrying capacity of the infant's red cells is reduced by 15–30 per cent, probably as a result of red-cell membrane damage.

Oxygen Saturation =

$$\frac{\text{(Oxygen content of sample } - \text{ oxygen in physical solution)}}{\text{(Oxygen capacity of sample } - \text{ oxygen in physical solution)}} \times 100 \text{ per cent.}$$

Normal Arterial Blood = Not less than 94 per cent saturated.

Normal Venous Blood = Approximately 70–90 per cent saturated (average value).

N.B.—Estimation of oxygen saturation of samples obtained at various sites during cardiac catheterization is useful when used in conjunction with intracardiac pressure measurements, in the detection of intracardiac abnormalities.

Fick Principle.—If the arteriovenous oxygen difference and total oxygen consumption over a timed period is known,

$$Cardiac\ Output =$$
$$\frac{\text{Total oxygen consumption per minute (ml./min.)}}{\text{Arteriovenous oxygen difference (ml.)}}$$

N.B.—During cardiac catheterization, the blood in the right auricle will give a good average venous sample: the blood from the lung periphery will give an oxygenated arterial sample.

REFERENCE.—Hawk, P. B., Oser, B. L., and Summerson, W. H. (1949), *Practical Physiological Chemistry*, 12th ed., 638. London: Churchill.

OXYTOCIN IN PLASMA

This estimation is not yet available.

ARTERIAL Po₂

Normal Values.—

Less than 30 years	90–100 mm. Hg	
30–40 years	85– 95 mm. Hg	With 95 per cent
40–60 years	75– 90 mm. Hg	saturation of
More than 60 years	65– 80 mm. Hg	hæmoglobin.
Breathing pure oxygen	610–670 mm. Hg	

Cyanosis is apparent when more than 5 g./100 ml. whole blood is in the form of reduced hæmoglobin, regardless of the total hæmoglobin concentration.

The normal alveolar ventilation=5–6 litres/min. Reduction of this ventilation rate by half reduces the Po_2 to 60 mm. Hg and causes hypoxæmia even though the hæmoglobin is 90 per cent saturated. When Po_2 falls to 40 mm. Hg this represents severe hypoxæmia, and when the Po_2 falls to 20 mm. Hg death occurs. The margin between cyanosis and fatal hypoxæmia is small.

Pathological.—
  Decrease.—
    1. *In newborn:*—
      Congenital malformations.
      Idiopathic respiratory distress syndrome.
      Pneumonia.
      Recurrent apnœa.
    2. *Children and adults:*—
      Pneumonia.
      Emphysema.
      Cardiac failure.
      Asthmatic bronchospasm. Falling Po_2 is accompanied by a rising Pco_2. If the Pco_2 falls towards normal values without improvement in the clinical condition or in the Po_2 the condition is very dangerous.
      Elderly patients in the early post-operative period.
      Low oxygen content of inspired air.

REFERENCES.—Davis, J. A. (1966), *Postgrad. Med. J.*, **42**, 386; Payne, J. P., and Conway, C. M. (1966), *Ibid.*, **42**, 341; McFadden, E. R., and Lyons, H. A. (1968), *New Engl. J. Med.*, **278**, 1027.

PANCREATIC ENZYME PROVOCATION TESTS

Theoretically, in chronic pancreatitis with partial or complete blockage of pancreatic ducts, and stimulation of surviving gland tissue, the secretion of amylase and lipase should pass into the blood-stream. The following substances, singly or in combination, have been tried unsuccessfully to demonstrate an abnormal rise in blood amylase and blood lipase:—

1. Secretin.
2. Morphine.
3. Bethanecol.
4. Methylcholine.

The author has also tried pancreozymin, and was unable to obtain consistent results. The study of duodenal juice obtained by intubation after the injection of secretin and pancreozymin may be useful in the differentiation of cases of steatorrhœa which are pancreatic in origin from other types.

N.B.—It has yet to be shown that provocative serum pancreatic enzyme tests serve any useful function in clinical practice.

REFERENCES.—Dreiling, D. A., and Richman, A. (1954), *Arch. intern. Med.*, **94**, 197 (67 references); Marks, I. N., and Tompsett, S. L. (1958), *Quart. J. Med.*, **27**, 431.

PARATHORMONE TOLERANCE TEST

Phosphate diuresis occurs in the 3 hours following intravenous or intramuscular injection of fresh parathormone extract (40–200 i.u.), especially if the initial urine phosphate excretion was low in:—

1. Normals.
2. Hypoparathyroidism.

After a low phosphate diet, the urine phosphate excretion increases to 50–180 mg./hour (as phosphate).

By contrast, there is no increase in urine phosphate excretion in pseudohypoparathyroidism after parathormone injection.

N.B.—It is important to check the potency of the hormone extract, by using a normal control at the same time as the test. When first introduced, normal cases did show a phosphate diuresis. The test is no longer reliable, since with the present-day hormone extract normal controls do not have a satisfactory phosphate diuresis.

REFERENCE.—Ellsworth, R., and Howard, J. E. (1934), *Bull. Johns Hopk. Hosp.*, **55**, 296.

PARATHYROID HORMONE IN PLASMA

Human parathyroid hormone, with a molecular weight of 9000–11,000, can be estimated in plasma by immuno-assay techniques. It has a very short half-life of approximately 20 minutes in the circulation. Normal daily production of the hormone in man is probably about 0·5–2 mg. There is a linear relationship between the parathyroid concentration and the plasma calcium concentration between plasma calcium values of 4 and 12 mg./100 ml. Hormone secretion is abolished when the plasma calcium level is 11–12 mg./100 ml.

Pathological.—

Increase.—

1. **Primary hyperparathyroidism.**—Raised serum calcium levels fail to depress hormone secretion.
2. **Ectopic hyperparathyroidism.**—The hormone may be released from ectopic tumours not of parathyroid origin, and not influenced by the serum calcium concentration.
3. **Secondary hyperparathyroidism.—**
    a. Chronic renal disease.
    b. Pseudohypoparathyroidism.
4. **Tertiary hyperparathyroidism.**—Following prolonged secondary hyperparathyroidism, there may develop autonomous hyperparathyroidism.

REFERENCES.—Potts, J. T., jun., Buckle, R. M., Sherwood, L. M., Ramberg, C. F., jun., Mayer, G. P., Kronfeld, O. S., Deftos, L. J., Cave, A. D., and Aurbach, G. D. (1968), *Parathyroid Hormone and Thyrocalcitonin (Calcitonin)*. Amsterdam: Excerpta Medica; Buckle, R. M. (1969), *Brit. med. J.*, **2**, 789.

*p*H OF CEREBROSPINAL FLUID

Fall in CSF *p*H is associated with disturbance of consciousness. Change in rate of respiration affects plasma *p*H, but does not affect CSF *p*H directly.

REFERENCE.—Posner, J. B., and Plum, F. (1967), *New Engl. J. Med.*, **277**, 605.

*p*H OF PLASMA (*Fig.* 2)

Normal Range.—*p*H = 7·37–7·42 in arterial blood.

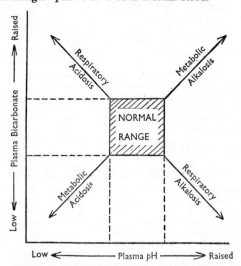

Fig. 2.—*p*H and bicarbonate in plasma.

N.B.—Arterialized venous blood can be obtained by warming the patient's hand in hot water (as hot as bearable), and puncturing a vein on the back of the hand with minimum stasis. The results obtained in this way agree well with arterial blood results (McGowan, G. K., 1959). In both compensated acidosis and alkalosis the plasma *p*H remains within the normal range. In severe metabolic and respiratory acidosis the plasma *p*H falls below 7·30 and in severe metabolic and respiratory alkalosis the plasma *p*H rises above 7·50. The extreme range of plasma *p*H found in disease which is still compatible with life is 6·95–7·80.

Pathological.—

1. *Alkalosis* (the plasma *p*H tends to rise):—

     a. Metabolic Alkalosis.—In this condition the plasma bicarbonate is raised:—
       i. Excessive alkali ingestion.
       ii. Greater loss of chloride relative to sodium, e.g., persistent vomiting or continuous gastric aspiration.
       iii. Potassium depletion.
       iv. Primary hyperaldosteronism.

     b. Respiratory Alkalosis.—In this condition the plasma bicarbonate is reduced.
       Over-ventilation.

2. *Acidosis* (the plasma *p*H tends to fall):—

     a. Metabolic Acidosis.—In this condition the plasma bicarbonate is reduced:—
       i. Starvation.
       ii. Ammonium chloride or calcium chloride ingestion.
       iii. Diabetes mellitus.
       iv. Severe diarrhœa.
       v. Renal failure.
       vi. Ureterocolic anastomosis.
       vii. Renal tubular acidosis.
       viii. Acute myocardial infarction.
       ix. Cyanotic congenital heart disease.

     b. Respiratory Acidosis.—In this condition the plasma bicarbonate is raised:—
       i. Emphysema.
       ii. Pneumonia.
       iii. Congestive cardiac failure with pulmonary congestion.
       iv. Progressive lung destruction.
       v. Morphine and associated drugs depress the respiratory centre.
       vi. Anæsthesia.

(*See also* ALKALI RESERVE IN PLASMA, p. 19.)

N.B.—Only in severe disturbances does the plasma *p*H fall outside the normal range. Small changes in *p*H are therefore significant. Unfortunately, these changes are technically difficult to detect. Very sensitive instruments and very careful collection of blood samples under paraffin are essential.

REFERENCE.—McGowan, G. K. (1959), personal communication.

pH OF URINE

Normal Range.—pH = 4·5–7·8. The normal maximum gradient against which renal tubules can transfer hydrogen ions is about 800 : 1, i.e., the urine pH lower limit is at pH 4·5 if the blood pH is 7·4.

There is no mechanism whereby a urine much more alkaline than the plasma can be secreted.

Following renal tubular damage, the hydrogen ion exchange mechanism and/or the ammonium excretion mechanism may be impaired, with resulting limitation in the urine pH range, and diminution in response of reaction to oral ammonium chloride or alkalis (Pitts, 1948).

Approaching pH 7·8, bicarbonate is excreted in the urine with base.

Approaching pH 4·5:—
1. Some free hydrogen ions derived from ionized carbonic acid are excreted.
2. The bulk of the urine phosphate is excreted in the form of monobase dihydrogen phosphate.

Urine Excretion of Acids.—
1. The urine pH falls towards 4·5.
2. The urine titratable acidity is increased (i.e., the sum of organic acids and sodium dihydrogen phosphate).
3. Ammonium ions are secreted by the distal renal tubules to combine with excess acid.

REFERENCE.—Pitts, R. F. (1948), *Fed. Proc.*, **7**, 418.

PHENOLSULPHTHALEIN EXCRETION TEST

After emptying the bladder, the patient drinks 600 ml. of water. Then dye solution (6 mg. of dye) is injected intravenously at the rate of 18 mg./m.² body surface area. If it is injected intravenously, 10 minutes are allowed for the dye to circulate. Urine is collected at 15, 30, 60, and 120 minutes.

Normal Results (expressed as percentage of dose excreted):—
1. *Individual Urine Samples*:—

15 min.	30 min.	60 min.	120 min.
28–51	31–24	9–17	3–10 per cent

2. *Total excreted after 1 Hour*: 40–60 per cent.
3. *Total excreted after 2 Hours*: 63–84 per cent.

The normal renal clearance of the dye is about 400 ml./min., i.e., 70 per cent may be excreted by the tubules, 30 per cent being filtered by the glomeruli. The inulin clearance (i.e., glomerular filtration rate) can be calculated from the result. In the presence of liver disease, the renal excretion rate is increased, since some of the dye is normally excreted by the liver in the bile.

REFERENCES.—Kasanen, A., and Kalliomaki, J. L. (1957), *Acta med. Scand.*, **159**, 341. (Review of 1000 tests); Healy, J. K. (1968), *Amer. J. Med.*, **44**, 348.

PHENYLKETONURIA. *See* **Amino-Acids** in Urine

PHOSPHATASE

ACID PHOSPHATASE IN SERUM.—The term "acid phosphatase" includes phosphomono-esterases which have an optimum *p*H of less than 7·0. The enzyme secreted by the prostate is formol stable and approximately the same fraction is alcohol labile. The normal non-prostatic serum acid phosphatase is carried by the platelets.

Physiological.—Serum total acid phosphatase is raised to twice the normal adult level at the second week of life, falling towards adult levels from 13 years to reach adult levels by 16–20 years, with no sex difference. L-Tartrate labile fraction remains at the same level in childhood as in adult life.

Serum Total Acid Phosphatase.—0·5–4·0 King-Armstrong units; up to 11 i.u./litre.

Serum Acid Phosphatase (Formol Stable).—0–2·0 King-Armstrong units; up to 4 i.u./litre.

Serum Acid Phosphatase (Tartrate Labile).—0–0·5 King-Armstrong units; up to 0·3 i.u./litre.

Pathological.—

Increase.—

1. *Formol Stable Fraction.*—(Copper stable, alcohol labile, L-tartrate labile.)

   Adult human prostate contains up to 1000 times the acid phosphatase of other tissues. This high acid phosphatase activity does not appear until puberty.

   Carcinoma of the Prostate.—The level may be abnormally raised, especially if the tumour has extended outside the gland. Anaplastic tumours tend not to secrete much, if any, enzyme.

   The serum level, after being raised in a case of carcinoma of the prostate, will fall:—

   a. Following successful removal of the tumour.

   b. Following effective œstrogen suppression of the tumour.

   c. Following a combination of (*a*) and (*b*).

   After successful treatment with œstrogens, if secondary deposits are present in the skeleton, the serum alkaline phosphatase, which will already be raised, increases still further as bone repair occurs, and then falls towards normal.

   In cases with liver secondary deposits, the serum alkaline phosphatase level, if raised, tends to fall rapidly, with regression of the secondaries.

2. *Total Serum Acid Phosphatase* (non-specific).—

   a. Carcinomatous bone deposits, especially from breast carcinoma. Levels above 5 units indicate active bone invasion.

   b. Paget's disease of bone, due to mobilization of bone acid phosphatase. (Very high serum alkaline phosphatase frequently found.)

   c. Hyperparathyroidism.

   d. Gaucher's disease (using disodium phenylphosphate as substrate, not inhibited by L-tartrate or copper salts).

   e. Following myocardial infarction or if platelets are destroyed excessively in the circulation the normal difference between serum and platelet-free heparinized plasma samples is reduced.

N.B.—**After prostatic massage, catheterization, or even after rectal examination, the serum acid phosphatase level (formol stable) is raised above normal for 24 hours.**

REFERENCES.—Herbert, F. K. (1946), *Quart. J. Med.*, **15**, 221; Abul-Fadl, M. A. M., and King, E. J. (1948), *J. clin. Path.*, **1**, 80; Jegatheesan, K. A., and Joplin, G. F. (1962), *Brit. med. J.*, **1**, 831.

ACID PHOSPHATASE IN URINE.

ACID PHOSPHATASE IN URINE.—In normal men, the first part of micturition washes out prostatic secretion and contains more acid phosphatase than the midstream fraction. The midstream fraction probably represents renal excretion of acid phosphatase. The final fraction contains more acid phosphatase, presumably derived from the prostate during straining.

Adult males before the sixth decade secrete more acid phosphatase than males after the sixth decade, whether the latter have carcinoma of the prostate or not.

Adult females with carcinoma of the breast and raised serum acid phosphatase levels secrete no more acid phosphatase than do normal women.

Normal Range.—
  Normal males (24–35 years old)—1462 King-Armstrong units/24 hr.
  Normal females (23–60 years old)—217 King-Armstrong units/24 hr.

REFERENCE.—Daniel, O., Kind, P. R. N., and King, E. J. (1954), *Brit. med. J.*, **1**, 19.

ALKALINE PHOSPHATASE IN SERUM.—

Normal Serum Range.—
  1. Birth—5–15 King-Armstrong units. Increased above normal in premature infants by 50–100 per cent.
  2. 1 month—10–30 King-Armstrong units.
  3. 3 years—10–20 King-Armstrong units.
  4. 10 years—15–30 King-Armstrong units.
  5. Adult—4·5–9·5 King-Armstrong units (50–150 i.u./litre).
  6. Senility—The levels are lower.

REFERENCE.—Philpot, G. R. (1968), *Proc. Assoc. Chim. Biochem.*, **5**, 48.

Physiological.—
  Increase.—
    The level is in the upper range of normal during the last 3 months of pregnancy, probably derived from the placenta. Normal levels are regained by 3–6 weeks post-partum.
  Decrease.—
    Apparently either inanition or a high protein diet may cause the serum alkaline phosphatase to fall into the lower range of normal.

Pathological.—
  Increase.—
    1. *Bone Metabolism.*—
      a. During the healing of a fracture.

b. Primary hyperparathyroidism
c. Secondary hyperparathyroidism
} only when the skeleton is overtly affected.

In primary hyperparathyroidism X-ray films show bone damage when the serum alkaline phosphatase exceeds 16 King-Armstrong unts.

Following removal of parathyroid tumour (*b*) the increased serum alkaline phosphatase level persists and may rise temporarily, falling gradually over a period of months as bone repair is completed.

d. Osteomalacia:—
   i. Low vitamin D in diet (rickets).
   ii. Calcium and/or phosphorus deficiency.
   iii. Steatorrhœa.
   iv. Chronic diarrhœa.
   v. Gastrocolic fistula.
   vi. Fanconi syndrome.
   vii. Renal tubular acidosis (Albright type). As Fanconi syndrome, but no amino-aciduria.
   viii. Partial gastrectomy. After this operation some cases show marked increase in serum alkaline phosphatase (some of which is derived from intestinal mucosa).

e. Paget's disease (osteitis deformans). Serum level gradually rises with extension of disease, rising rapidly if osteogenic sarcoma develops. ACTH or cortisone causes a transitory fall, often followed by a sharp rebound increase.

Osteoporosis circumscripta of skull, related to Paget's disease, is also associated with a raised serum level.

f. Cushing's syndrome (presumably due to excess ACTH).

g. Osteosclerosis fragilitas generalisata (marble bone).

h. Some cases of polyostotic fibrous dysplasia.

i. Hereditary hyperphosphatasæmia. Rapid turnover of lamellar bone with failure to lay down compact cortical bone. Skeletal and skull defects result.

N.B.—In bone disease the serum glutamic-oxalacetic transaminase is not increased.

  2. *Renal Disease.*—"Renal rickets". Due to vitamin D resistant rickets associated with secondary hyperparathyroidism.

  3. *Bone Damage.*—
    a. Metastatic carcinoma in bone.
    b. Osteogenic sarcoma. Removal of tumour results in a sharp fall in serum enzyme level, with increase as metastases appear. In predominantly osteolytic forms the serum level remains normal or only moderately increased.
    c. Myeloma. A slight rise may occur in some cases.
    d. Hodgkin's disease, if the bones are invaded.
    e. Gaucher's disease, with bone resorption.

REFERENCES.—Woodward, H. O., and Craven, L. F. (1940), *J. clin. Invest.*, **19**, 1; Dent, C. E., and Harper, C. M. (1962), *Lancet*, **1**, 559; Birkett, D. J., Done, J., Neale, F. C., and Posen, S. (1966), *Brit. med. J.*, **1**, 1211; Thompson, R. C., jun., Gaull, G. E., Horowitz, S. J., and Schenk, R. K. (1969), *Amer. J. Med.*, **47**, 209.

N.B.—Osteoporosis has no influence on the serum alkaline phosphatase.

4. *Infectious Mononucleosis.*—Serum level increased in many cases, with maximum values during the third week of the disease.

    i. Hepatic disorders. Uncomplicated extrahepatic biliary obstruction. The serum level tends to be greater than 30 units. Liver iso-enzyme is induced.

    ii. Cytomegalovirus infection in infants.

    iii. Cholangitis and cholangiolitis.

    iv. Hepatocellular jaundice. The serum levels are most commonly between 12 and 30 units.

    v. Portal cirrhosis. Increases in some cases.

    vi. Secondary carcinoma, liver abscess, echinococcus cyst, and sarcoidosis, involving the liver, may all increase the serum level.

    vii. Active liver regeneration.

    viii. Active bile-duct proliferation.

    ix. Liver abscess.

5. Extrahepatic sepsis.

REFERENCES.—Neale, G., Caughey, D. E., Mollin, D. L., and Booth, C. C. (1966), *Brit. med. J.*, **1**, 382; Kaplan, M. M., and Righetti, Adriana (1969), *J. clin. Invest.*, **48**, 42a.

N.B.—Congenital bile-duct atresia and also hæmolytic jaundice have no effect on the serum alkaline phosphatase levels. On the other hand, the serum glutamic-oxalacetic transaminase is increased in liver disease.

Decrease.—

1. Hypophosphatasæmia. A possibly hereditary infantile condition showing defective bone calcification, normal serum calcium and plasma inorganic phosphate, but very low bone and serum alkaline phosphatase activity.

2. Hypothyroidism.

3. Scurvy.

4. Gross anæmia.

5. Kwashiorkor.

    Following treatment there is a further fall in the first 2 weeks, followed by a rise to normal levels.

6. Achondroplasia.

    Following arrest of growth in childhood, serum level falls rapidly to adult levels.

7. Cretinism.

    Following arrest of growth, serum level falls rapidly to normal adult levels.

8. Deposit of radioactive materials in bone results in low serum enzyme levels, presumably results from damage to osteoblasts.

    Study of iso-enzyme components of alkaline phosphatase is promising and enables iso-enzymes in (*a*) bone disorders, (*b*) liver disorders, (*c*) intestinal alkaline phosphatase in Laennec's cirrhosis, to be distinguished.

9. Patients on clofibrate therapy.

REFERENCES.—King, E. J. (1956), *Micro-analysis in Medical Bio-chemistry*, 3rd ed. London: Churchill; Gutman, A. B. (1959), *Amer. J. Med.*, **27**, 875 (review with 355 references); Kaplan, M. M., and Rogers, L. (1969), *Lancet*, **2**, 1029; Smith, A. F., MacFie, W. G., and Oliver, M. F. (1970), *Brit. med. J.*, **1**, 86.

ALKALINE PHOSPHATASE IN SYNOVIAL FLUID.—Synovial fluid alkaline phosphatase activity is normally greater than the corresponding serum level.

Pathological.—

Decrease.—Pseudo-gout.

REFERENCES.—Davies, D. V. (1969), in *Textbook of the Rheumatic Diseases* (Ed. Copeman, W. S. C.), London: Livingstone; Yaron, M., Yust, I., and Zurkowski, P. (1969), *Lancet*, **2**, 651.

ALKALINE PHOSPHATASE IN URINE.—

Normal Range.—

Males—up to 6000 units ⎱ In 8-hr. overnight urine
Females—up to 7560 units ⎰ sample.

Pathological.—

Increase.—

1. Acute glomerular nephritis.
2. Nephritis associated with lupus erythematosus.
3. Diabetic nephrosclerosis.

REFERENCE.—Amador, E., Dorfman, L. E., and Wacker, L. E. C. (1965), *Ann. intern. Med.*, **62**, 30.

GLUCOSE-6-PHOSPHATASE IN SERUM.—

The enzyme catalyses the reaction:—

Glucose-6-phosphate $\rightleftharpoons$ Glucose + free phosphate.

The enzyme is present in liver, and normally is present in serum in very low concentrations only.

Normal Range.—0–12 units/ml.

Pathological.—

Increase.—

1. *Hepatitis.*—After liver damage with carbon tetrachloride the serum level reaches its peak values by 6 hours (cf. later rise of SGOT and SGPT).
2. *Cirrhosis.*—Moderate rise described.
3. *Renal Disease.*—Slight rise.

N.B.—Hæmolysis invalidates serum estimation because of high red-cell content of non-specific phosphatases.

REFERENCE.—Koide, H., and Oda, T. (1959), *Clin. chim. Acta*, **4**, 554.

PHOSPHATE

INORGANIC PHOSPHATE IN PLASMA.—

Normal Range.—

At birth—4·0–8·5 mg./100 ml. (2·4–5·0 mEq./litre).
1 week—4·0–7·0 mg./100 ml. (2·4–4·1 mEq./litre).
6 years—3·5–5·5 mg./100 ml. (2·1–3·2 mEq./litre).
15 years—3·5–4·5 mg./100 ml. (2·1–2·6 mEq./litre).
Adult—3·0–4·5 mg./100 ml. (1·8–2·6 mEq./litre).

$$\left(\frac{\text{mg./litre}}{30\cdot9} = \text{mmol./litre.} \right)$$

REFERENCE.—King, E. J. (1932), *Biochem. J.*, **26**, 292.

Physiological.—During carbohydrate utilization (i.e., after a carbohydrate meal) phosphate and potassium enter the cells with glucose. Blood for inorganic phosphate estimation should therefore be taken from fasting patients. The presence of phosphatase and organic phosphates in the red cells necessitates rapid separation of plasma or serum, or otherwise a false high reading for the inorganic phosphate is obtained.

Pathological.—
Increase.—
1. Vitamin-D excess.
2. Healing fractures.
X 3. Renal failure (with associated sulphate retention).
4. Hypoparathyroidism.
5. Pseudohypoparathyroidism.
6. Diabetic ketosis.
7. Acromegaly.
8. Newborn infants fed on unadapted cow's milk, which has a much higher phosphate content than human milk.
9. Malignant hyperpyrexia following anæsthesia.

Decrease.—
1. Hyperinsulinism. During successful treatment of diabetic ketosis, insulin causes phosphate ions to enter the cells with glucose and potassium.
2. Hyperparathyroidism. Parathyroid hormone causes a marked phosphaturia.
3. Osteomalacia, e.g., childhood rickets.
4. Steatorrhœa (low vitamin-D absorption from small bowel).
5. Fanconi's syndrome and Albright's type of renal acidosis (gross phosphaturia).
6. Hypopituitarism with growth hormone deficiency in children.
7. Acute alcoholism.
8. Gram-negative bacterial septicæmia (<2 mg. per cent).
9. Associated with hypokalæmia.

N.B.—**In normal individuals undergoing glucose tolerance tests, the plasma inorganic phosphate runs an inverse curve to the blood-sugar readings. The curve is flattened in diabetics.**

REFERENCES.—Stein, J. H., Smith, W. O., and Ginn, H. E. (1966), *Amer. J. med. Sci.*, **252**, 78; Oppé, T. E., and Redstone, D. (1968), *Lancet*, **1**, 1045; Anderson, D. C., Peters, T. J., and Stewart, W. K. (1969), *Brit. med. J.*, **4**, 402; Riedler, G. F., and Scheitlin, W. A. (1969), *Ibid.*, **1**, 753.

INORGANIC PHOSPHATE IN URINE.—

Normal Output.—0·5–1·5 g./24 hr. (as phosphorus). The output varies widely, depending on the diet. Even with careful balance studies, phosphate metabolism is difficult to interpret.

Pathological.—
Increase.—
1. Hyperparathyroidism.
2. Avitaminosis D, on adequate dietary phosphate and low calcium intake.
3. "Vitamin-D resistant" rickets.

4. Lignac-Fanconi syndrome.
5. Renal acidosis:—
    a. Lightwood-Butler type shows no increase.
    b. Albright type shows an increase.
6. Normal person (especially a child) immobilized following paraplegia, or a fracture.
7. Vitamin-D intoxication.
8. Non-renal acidosis (increased phosphate excretion as a urine buffer).

Decrease.—
1. Hypoparathyroidism.
2. Parathyroidectomy.
3. Pseudohypoparathyroidism.
4. Avitaminosis D on high calcium intake. Insoluble calcium phosphate is excreted in the stools.

PHOSPHATE IN FÆCES.—

Normal Output.—On a normal balanced diet containing 1–2 g. of phosphorus, the fæcal output ranges from 0·4 to 0·8 g./24 hr. It consists of both organic and inorganic phosphate.

Increased Output.—
1. Vitamin-D deficiency (if there is adequate dietary phosphate).
2. Administration of aluminium hydroxide. (This may be given to slow down the rate of formation of renal phosphate-containing calculi.)
3. Steatorrhœa, from any cause (i.e., absorption of phosphorus is impeded).

Decreased Output.—Vitamin-D intoxication (i.e., excessive absorption of phosphate).

N.B.—**The estimation of fæcal phosphate is useful only in specialized balance studies.**

PHOSPHOGLUCOMUTASE IN SERUM

The enzyme catalyses the reaction:—

Glucose-1-phosphate ⇌ Glucose-6-phosphate.

The enzyme is widely distributed throughout the body tissues.

Normal Range.—4–17 i.u./litre. (The day-to-day fluctuation in any single subject is wide.)

Red blood-cells contain the enzyme in concentrations higher than the normal serum level. Therefore avoid hæmolysis.

Pathological.—
Increase.—
1. Acute hepatitis.
2. Carcinoma. It has been used to measure the response in carcinomatosis to pituitary ablation, but is not as useful for this as is the estimation of serum phosphohexose-isomerase.
3. Leukæmia. Increases in some cases.
4. Carbon monoxide poisoning. 1 case with serum level increased 250 × normal reported.

There would appear to be no special indication for estimating this enzyme at present, in clinical practice.

REFERENCES.—Noltmann, E., and Bruns, F. H. (1958), *Hoppe-Seyl. Z.*, **313**, 194; Joplin, G. F., and Jegatheesan, K. A. (1962), *Brit. med. J.*, **1**, 827.

PHOSPHOHEXOSEISOMERASE IN SERUM

The enzyme catalyses the reaction:—

$$Glucose\text{-}6\text{-}phosphate \rightleftharpoons Fructose\text{-}6\text{-}phosphate.$$

The highest tissue concentrations are found in liver and skeletal muscle ($1000 \times$ normal serum level). Red blood-cells contain the enzyme at $100 \times$ the normal serum level, and therefore hæmolysis invalidates the estimation. The enzyme is also present in kidney, heart, and brain.

Normal Range.— 8–40 units (Bodansky).

Pathological.—
Increase.—

1. *Progressive Muscular Atrophy.*
2. *Hepatitis.*—In homologous serum jaundice and infective hepatitis the serum level rises rapidly in the early stages, falling to normal by the third and fourth weeks. Experimental toxic hepatitis causes a marked rise in serum levels.
3. *Cirrhosis.*—Normal or slightly raised levels found.
4. *Biliary Obstruction.*—Normal or slightly raised levels found.
5. *Myocardial Infarction.*—Serum levels increase by 6–12 hours, reaching a peak by 24–48 hours, which is from 2–15 × normal, falling to normal by 4–7 days.
6. *Carcinoma.*—
   a. In carcinoma of the prostate high values are found, which are roughly parallel with the serum acid phosphatase values.
   b. In carcinoma of the breast high values are found, especially when there are metastases.
   c. Carcinomatosis. High values are found, especially when there are bone secondaries. This estimation has been successfully used to assess response to treatment designed to produce a remission, e.g., pituitary ablation.
7. *Hæmolytic Anæmia.*—Presumably the enzyme is released from breaking down red cells.
8. *Acute and Chronic Myeloid Leukæmia.*—The serum level rises and falls with the white blood-cell count. The serum level is partially derived from breaking down neutrophils (which contain at least twice as much PHI as do lymphocytes).
9. *Megaloblastic Anæmia.*—Serum levels rise to up to $9 \times$ normal. The estimation of PHI is probably most useful in assessing cases of carcinoma in relation to treatment.

REFERENCES.—Bodansky, O. (1954), *Cancer*, **7**, 1200 and 1191; Bruns, F. H., and Jacob, W. (1954), *Klin. Wschr.*, **32**, 1041; Israels, L. G., Delory, G. E., Hnatiuk, L., and Friesen, E. (1958), *Blood*, **13**, 79.

PHOSPHOHEXOSEISOMERASE IN VAGINAL FLUID

Vaginal fluid aspirates derived from the adult female cervix have been studied in an attempt to screen women for the presence of early carcinoma.

While raised levels are found in cases with carcinoma of the cervix, "false negative" results may occur in cases with carcinoma-in-situ, and "false positive" results are obtained in the presence of vaginal infection or bleeding. This enzyme estimation appears to be better than either glucose-6-phosphate dehydrogenase or 6-phosphogluconate dehydrogenase.

REFERENCES.—Cameron, C. B., and Husain, O. A. N. (1965), *Brit. med. J.*, 1, 1529; Muir, G. M. (1966), *J. clin. Path.*, 19, 378.

PIGMENT

PIGMENT IN CEREBROSPINAL FLUID.—

Xanthochromia occurs in:—
1. Post-hæmorrhage. The yellow tint is apparent in the supernatant fluid within a few hours of a hæmorrhage. In the absence of further hæmorrhage it disappears within 3–4 weeks.
2. Severe meningitis ⎱ Presumably some oozing of blood
3. Brain abscess ⎰ occurs from the inflamed areas.
4. Stasis below a block. There is frequently a raised fibrinogen concentration and the albumin/globulin ratio is increased in the fluid.
5. Jaundice. Bilirubin tinges the cerebrospinal fluid.
6. Dyes, e.g., acriflavin.

N.B.—Xanthochromia has been associated with an elevated glutamine content of the cerebrospinal fluid. This is thought to be due to an overall increase in amino-acids. The cause remains unknown.

REFERENCE.—Scott, T. G. (1958), *Clin. chim. Acta*, 3, 343.

PIGMENTS IN URINE.—

Normal.—The normal amber-yellow tint in urine is due to urochrome. This substance appears to be excreted in amounts proportional to the metabolic rate.

Uro-erythrin appears as a pink pigment present on uric acid and urate deposits.

Normal urine is nearly colourless when large volumes of fluid are ingested. Conversely it becomes deeply orange-brown following dehydration. On standing, urine becomes cloudy when the reaction is alkaline, as the phosphates precipitate.

Abnormal.—
1. *Orange*:—
   a. Urobilin in excess.
   b. Eosin (green fluorescence).
   c. Santonin.
   d. Pyridium.
   e. Crysophanic acid.
2. *Red*:—
   a. Blood-pigments, including myoglobin.
   b. Porphyrins.
   c. Amidopyrine.
   d. Pyridium.
   e. Aniline dyes in sweets.
   f. Madder. A dye used in foods.
   g. Fuchsine. A dye used in foods.
   h. Bilberries.

i. Beetroot. Anthrocyaninuria, inherited via a recessive Mendelian character.
3. *Purple-red:*—
    a. Phenolphthalein
    b. Phenol red $\Big\}$ In alkaline urine.
4. *Red-brown to Dark Brown:*—
    a. Methæmoglobin.
    b. Porphyrins.
    c. Phenolic drug poisoning.
5. *Brown-black:*—
    a. Melanin.
    b. Homogentisic acid (alkaptonuria).
    c. Excessive amounts of hæmoglobin on standing.
    d. Lysol and carbolic acid poisoning.
6. *Green-blue:*—
    a. Methylene blue.
    b. Biliverdin.
    c. Pyocyaneus infection (or contamination of sample).
    d. Indicans (intestinal putrefaction, carbolic poisoning).
7. *Green-yellow:*—
    a. Bile-pigments.
8. *Yellow:*—
    a. Mepacrine.
    b. Furadantin.
    c. Riboflavin in large doses.
9. *Brown-yellow in Acid Urine, turning Red with Alkali:*—
    a. Senna.
    b. Rhubarb.
    c. Chelidonium.
    d. Dindevan.
10. *Milky Urine:*—
    a. Infection (pus cells and bacteria).
    b. Chyluria.

PORPHYRINS

The term "porphyrin" embraces the series of pigments related to hæmoglobin, and which may be produced either during its synthesis or during its breakdown. Chemically they are cyclic tetrapyrrolic in nature, thus revealing their relationship to hæm and its homologues. Iron is absent from the molecule. In man they exist in two series, Series I and Series III: hæmoglobin is formed only from Series III porphyrins and their precursor, porphobilinogen.

Normally, as a result of hæmoglobin synthesis and breakdown small amounts of porphyrins appear in both the urine and the stool.

Pathological.—Those diseases which are associated with primary abnormality of porphyrin synthesis are referred to as *Porphyrias*.

There are many conditions in which porphyrin synthesis is interfered with secondarily, with a moderate increase in porphyrin excretion. These conditions are grouped together as acquired *Porphyrinurias*.

REFERENCE.—Gray, C. H. (1970), in *Biochemical Disorders in Human Disease*, 3rd ed. (Ed. Thompson, R. H. S., and Wootton, I. D. P.). London: Churchill.

Δ-AMINO LÆVULINIC ACID IN URINE.—

Normal Output.—Up to 2 mg./day.

Pathological Increase.—

1. Acute intermittent porphyria.
2. Porphyria variegata (acute).
3. Hexachlorobenzene porphyria.
4. Lead poisoning.

COPROPORPHYRIN IN ERYTHROCYTES.—

Normal Range.—1–2·5 μg./100 ml. red cells.

Pathological.—

Increase.—

1. Erythropoietic porphyria.
2. Erythropoietic protoporphyria.
3. Erythropoietic coproporphyria.
4. Griseofulvin porphyria.

COPROPORPHYRIN IN FÆCES.—

Normal Output.—0–20 μg./g. dry weight. Up to 400 μg./24 hr.

1. Fæcal coproporphyrin is probably normally related to the amount of meat in the diet.
2. Chemically induced hæmolytic anæmia leads to an increased excretion of coproporphyrin III in the fæces.
3. Erythropoietic porphyria.
4. Acute intermittent porphyria (slight).
5. Porphyria variegata, acute and chronic (slight).
6. Erythropoietic protoporphyria (variable).
7. Erythropoietic coproporphyria.
8. Symptomatic hepatic cutaneous porphyria.
9. Griseofulvin porphyria.

COPROPORPHYRIN IN URINE.—

Normal Output.—60–280 μg./24 hr. (60–80 per cent Series I). (Urine output increased in alkaline urine).

Pathological.—

Increase.—

1. Erythropoietic porphyria.
2. Acute intermittent porphyria (slight increase).
3. Porphyria variegata (acute). Variable increase in chronic state.
4. Symptomatic hepatic cutaneous porphyria (slight increase).
5. Bantu porphyria.
6. Hexachlorobenzene porphyria.
7. Viral hepatitis. There may also be increased amounts of porphobilinogen and uroporphyrin I in the urine.
8. Acute infections. Up to 500 μg./24 hr. may be excreted.
9. Phenylhydrazine poisoning.
10. Hæmolytic anæmia ⎫ i.e., increased hæmopoiesis.
11. Polycythæmia vera ⎭
12. Moderate increase in pernicious anæmia.
13. Heavy metal poisoning. In lead poisoning an increase in urine coproporphyrin III is associated with an increase in urine uroporphyrin and red-cell protoporphyrin.
14. Refractory anæmia (aplastic).
15. Portal cirrhosis. There may also be an increase in urine uroporphyrin I and porphobilinogen.

16. Acute poliomyelitis. Possibly it is derived from the central nervous system.
17. Pseudohypertrophic muscular dystrophy.
18. Pellagra.
19. Intoxication with:—
    a. Alcohol.
    b. Antipyretics.
    c. Barbiturates.
    d. Organic arsenical compounds.
    e. Sulphonamides.
20. Acute rheumatic fever.
21. Severe iron-deficiency anæmia.
22. Heavy ethyl alcohol ingestion.
23. Burns cases.

N.B.—The amount of porphyrin excreted in induced porphyrinuria is not as large as in the idiopathic and congenital porphyrias, e.g., lead poisoning—usually less than 5 mg./24 hr.; other non-porphyrias—less than 1 mg./24 hr.

PORPHYRIN IN PLASMA.—
Normal.—Not detectable in plasma.
Pathological.—
  Increase.—
    1. Erythropoietic porphyria.
    2. Porphyria variegata (acute).
    3. Erythropoietic protoporphyria.
    4. Erythropoietic coproporphyria.
    5. Symptomatic hepatic cutaneous porphyria (during liver dysfunction).
    6. Griseofulvin porphyria.

PORPHOBILINOGEN IN FÆCES.—Porphobilinogen does not appear normally in the stool.

PORPHOBILINOGEN IN URINE.—
Normal Output.—1–1·5 mg./24 hr.
Pathological.—
  Increase.—
    1. *Acute Intermittent Porphyria.*—Up to 50 mg. of porphobilinogen may be excreted in the urine daily during an acute attack. Increased quantities of uroporphyrin I and coproporphyrin I also appear in the urine.
    2. *Liver Disease.*—A slight increase in urine porphobilinogen may occur in liver disease, probably due to deviation of normal porphyrin excretion via the bile to the urine.
    3. *Porphyria Variegata* (acute).
    4. Hexachlorobenzene porphyria.
    5. Patients treated with promazine excrete a metabolite which gives a false-positive urine test for porphobilinogen.
       Porphobilinogen forms a red colour when treated with a solution of acid paradimethylaminobenzaldehyde. After buffering with sodium acetate, the colour intensifies and is not extractable by chloroform. The finding of increased porphobilinogen in urine on qualitative testing is virtually pathognomonic of acute

idiopathic porphyria, or porphyria cutanea tarda. The diagnosis should be confirmed by demonstrating porphyrins in excess.

PROTOPORPHYRIN IN ERYTHROCYTES.—
Normal Range.—10–60 μg./100 ml. red cells.
Pathological.—
Increase.—
1. Erythropoietic porphyria.
2. Erythropoietic protoporphyria (marked increase).
3. Griseofulvin porphyria.
4. Iron-deficiency anæmia.

PROTOPORPHYRIN IN FÆCES.—
Normal Output.—0–30 μg./g. dry weight. Up to 955 μg./day.
1. Porphyria variegata (acute and chronic).
2. Erythropoietic protoporphyria.
3. Griseofulvin porphyria.
4. Symptomatic hepatic cutaneous porphyria (normal or slight increase).

UROPORPHYRIN IN ERYTHROCYTES.—
Normal Range.—Traces only.
Pathological.—
Increase.—Erythropoietic porphyria.

UROPORPHYRIN IN FÆCES.—
Normal Output.—Up to 50 μg./24 hr.
Pathological.—
Increase.—
1. Erythropoietic porphyria.
2. Acute intermittent porphyria.
3. Porphyria variegata (chronic phase).

UROPORPHYRIN IN URINE.—
Normal Output.—5–30 μg. per 24 hours, mainly Series I.
Pathological.—
Increase.—
1. Erythropoietic porphyria.
2. Porphyria variegata, in acute attacks (variable excretion in chronic phase).
3. Symptomatic hepatic cutaneous porphyria.
4. Hexachlorobenzene porphyria.
5. Acute intermittent porphyria (variable).
6. Some cases of portal cirrhosis.

POTASSIUM

POTASSIUM IN CEREBROSPINAL FLUID.—This estimation is of no clinical importance. The concentration in cerebrospinal fluid is approximately 70 per cent of the plasma level.

POTASSIUM IN FÆCES.—
Normal Output.—Approximately 5 mEq./24 hr. In severe diarrhœa 60 mEq. or more of potassium may be lost in the stools per day. The accurate measurement of fæcal potassium is usual only in metabolic balance studies.

In clinical practice this source of potassium loss should be remembered, particularly in infants who are unable to withstand imbalances in water and electrolytes to the same degree as adults.

Fæcal potassium grossly increased following secretion by villous tumours of colon and rectum.

REFERENCE.—Roy, A. D., and Ellis, H. (1959), *Lancet*, **1**, 759.

POTASSIUM IN GASTRIC JUICE.—

Normal Concentration.—10 mEq./litre (mmol./litre). (Parietal and non-parietal juice have the same potassium concentration.)

Pathological.—

Increase.—Associated with damage to the gastric mucous membrane.

POTASSIUM IN PLASMA.—

Normal Range.—

Males.—Mean = 4 mEq./litre (mmol./litre). Range = 3·5–4·5 mEq./litre (mmol./litre).

Females.—Mean = 3·9 mEq./litre (mmol./litre). Range = 3·4–4·4 mEq./litre (mmol./litre).

REFERENCE.—Flynn, F. V. (1969), *Ann. Clin. Biochem.*, **6**, 1.

It has been shown, using radioactive potassium, that injected potassium equilibrates in the extracellular fluid within a few minutes, whereas it equilibrates with the intracellular fluid in about 15 hours. The plasma concentration of potassium is a function of the rapidity of its removal by the kidneys. Therefore the serum potassium concentration can be independent, at least temporarily, of the potassium store in the body cells, e.g.:—

1. In metabolic alkalosis with good renal function there is usually potassium deficiency with low plasma potassium concentration.

2. In metabolic alkalosis with poor renal function there is potassium deficiency, but the plasma potassium level is normal or elevated.

Thus, the interpretation of plasma potassium values must always be made after careful assessment of the clinical condition of the patient.

Pathological.—

Increase.—(Increase in plasma potassium occurs when there is both excessive intake of potassium or liberation of cell potassium, and also renal insufficiency.)—

1. *Contraction of Volume of Extracellular Fluid.*—The plasma potassium is frequently increased in shock states, especially if accompanied by metabolic acidosis; but the conditions causing shock are associated with renal insufficiency and/or liberation of cell potassium.

2. *Transfer of Potassium from Intracellular to Extracellular Fluid.—*

   a. Massive hæmolysis results in release of red-cell potassium. In the presence of renal failure the plasma level rises rapidly.

   b. Anuria from any cause.

   c. Crush syndrome and other forms of tissue ischæmia. There is release of potassium from muscle cells, and also often associated renal failure.

   d. Hyperkinetic activity. For example in status epilepticus, or strychnine poisoning, the plasma potassium increases, especially if the extracellular fluid is reduced, as occurs in dehydration.

  e. Malignant hyperpyrexia following anæsthesia.

  f. Hyperkalæmic periodic paralysis. Attacks occur especially 30–40 minutes after exercise.

3. *Reduced Renal Excretion.*—

  a. Addison's disease. There is reduced potassium excretion in the urine, with increased sodium loss, and progressive rise in the plasma potassium level.

  b. Renal failure. Potassium is liberated during body cell breakdown, and is not excreted completely in the urine.

  c. Diabetic ketosis. There is impaired uptake of potassium by the cells, and increased liberation of cell potassium following protein breakdown and gluconeogenesis.

4. *Rapid Administration of Potassium.*—Even in the presence of gross cell potassium deficiency, rapid infusion of potassium salts can cause a marked rise in the plasma potassium concentration, and can lead to cardiac arrest.

N.B.—Patients with potassium deficiency and an associated metabolic alkalosis or raised plasma sodium level are less likely to suffer from potassium intoxication following infusion of potassium salts.

Spurious elevated serum potassium levels may be obtained on occasion.

  a. Exercise of arm with occlusive cuff in place.

  b. Hæmolysis of blood sample, or delay in separation of plasma from red cells.

  c. Release of potassium from platelets during clotting, if serum used.

Decrease.—

1. *Inadequate Intake of Potassium.*—After operations on the gastro-intestinal tract, in œsophageal stricture, or with upper intestinal obstruction, for example, intake of potassium may be grossly reduced.

2. *Excessive Loss of Potassium from the Gastro-intestinal Tract.*—Prolonged vomiting, fistulæ, steatorrhœa, or severe diarrhœa cause abnormally large amounts of potassium to be lost.

3. *Excessive Loss of Potassium in the Urine.*—

  a. In diabetic ketosis potassium is liberated from the cells during gluconeogenesis. Much of this potassium is excreted in the urine combined with the ketone bodies.

  b. Hormone action:—

    i. The administration of ACTH causes potassium loss in the urine with sodium retention. Increased dietary sodium chloride increases this loss.

    ii. DOCA administration causes sodium retention and potassium loss in the urine.

    iii. Cortisone (if more than 100 mg./day), adrenal extract, corticosterone, 17-hydroxycorticosterone, may all produce potassium deficiency.

iv. In Cushing's syndrome there is excessive endogenous adrenocortical activity with increased potassium loss in the urine.

v. In liver disease and also in congestive cardiac failure, it is possible that the liver may be unable to catabolize adrenal steroids at a normal rate. Hence normally secreted steroids would then overact.

vi. Hyperaldosteronism results in gross urine potassium loss.

c. Carbenoxolone therapy.

4. *Diuretic Action.—*

a. Organic mercurial diuretics may cause excessive excretion of potassium with chloride in the urine.

b. Acetazolamide, by inhibiting the formation of bicarbonate ions in the renal tubular cells, increases the loss of potassium in the urine.

c. Para-aminosalicylate therapy increases the urine potassium loss.

5. *Renal Disease.—*

a. In renal tubular acidosis, hydrogen ion and ammonium ion production by the renal tubule cells is diminished, with excessive loss of potassium in the urine. In any case of severe renal damage, potassium conservation may be impaired.

b. Bartter's syndrome.

6. *Transfer of Potassium from the Extracellular Fluid to the Intracellular Fluid.—*

a. Diabetic ketosis treated with insulin. Potassium passes into the cells with glucose when insulin is given. After prolonged ketosis there is a large potassium deficit and a marked fall in the plasma potassium level may occur.

b. Testosterone therapy causes increased protein anabolism and hence promotes the transfer of potassium into the cells, with phosphate.

c. It is thought that sudden attacks of paralysis in familial periodic paralysis are presaged by a gross transfer of potassium into the intracellular fluid.

7. *Dilution of Extracellular Potassium.—*Prolonged administration of potassium-poor fluids results in a low plasma potassium, when no additional potassium salts or potassium-containing foods are being taken by mouth, e.g., post-operative states.

POTASSIUM IN RED BLOOD-CELLS.—

Normal Range.—77–87 mEq./litre packed cells.

Pathological.—

Decrease.—

1. Long-term diuretic therapy.
2. Aldosteronism.

REFERENCE.—Boyd, D. W. (1970), *Lancet*, **1**, 594.

POTASSIUM IN URINE.—

Normal Output.—1·4–3·5 g. (35–90 mEq.)/24 hr. The amount varies with the dietary intake.

In the presence of adequate body potassium, ingested potassium is excreted in the urine in about 4 hours. This is the basis for the potassium tolerance test which has been used in the past for the detection of mild hypoadrenalism (early Addison's disease); in fact, the test is far too dangerous and uncertain for clinical use (Zwermer and Truszkowski, 1937).

Potassium is filtered freely by the glomeruli and reabsorbed by the proximal tubules. Potassium secretion (passive diffusion following active sodium reabsorption) occurs in the distal tubules.

Normal adults, when deprived of a normal potassium intake, continue to excrete 20–50 mEq. of potassium per 24 hours in the urine for 3–4 days before the excretion rate falls. On an electrolyte-free diet containing carbohydrate and fat only, the urine potassium falls to 10 mEq./24 hr. after 48 hr.

In the presence of sodium deficiency, potassium from the intracellular space passes into the extracellular fluid. Potassium is then preferentially secreted in the urine, sodium being retained (Lowe, 1953).

Pathological.—

Decrease.—

1. Renal disease with low urine flow:—
    a. Severe acute glomerulonephritis.
    b. Pyelonephritis.
    c. Terminal nephrosclerosis.
    d. "Salt-losing nephritis".
2. Extra-renal uræmia, with oliguria.
3. Addison's disease.
4. Chronic potassium depletion without gross sodium deficiency, e.g., after prolonged diarrhœa, purgative addicts. Urine output, both of sodium and potassium, are low.

Increase.—

1. Steroid hormone action:—
    a. Administration of:—
        i. ACTH.
        ii. DOCA.
        iii. Hydrocortisone.
        iv. Cortisone.
    b. Cushing's syndrome.
    c. Primary hyperaldosteronism.

In these conditions excess potassium is excreted in the urine and sodium is retained. Sodium chloride administration exaggerates this.

2. Renal disease:—
    a. Renal tubule acidosis (Albright type).
    b. Fanconi syndrome.
    c. Diuretic recovery phase of acute tubular necrosis.
    d. Potassium-losing nephritis.

3. Diuretics:—
    a. Carbonic anhydrase inhibitor impairs hydrogen ion exchange for potassium in the renal tubules, even in the absence of diuresis. Increased excretion of bicarbonate ions causes increased potassium excretion.

   b. Organic mercurial diuretics cause potassium excretion
      by increasing the urine volume, potassium ions dif-
      fusing passively into the tubular fluid.
4. Metabolic acidosis, e.g., diabetes mellitus, in which
   potassium is excreted with the excess organic acids.
5. Metabolic alkalosis, e.g., prolonged vomiting, or excessive intake of sodium bicarbonate.
6. Starvation, i.e., increased breakdown of the body cells
   occurs, with release of intracellular potassium. Carbohydrate intake (glucose 100 g./24 hr.) greatly reduces
   the rate of cell breakdown.

N.B.—**Administration of sodium chloride to potassium
depleted patients will cause a further loss of potassium in the
urine.**

REFERENCES.—Zwermer, R. L., and Truszkowski, T. (1937), *Biochem.
    J.*, **31**, 229; Lowe, K. G. (1953), *Clin. Sci.*, **12**, 57.

PREGNANEDIOL IN URINE

Range in Normal Pregnancy.—
   1st trimester—rises from 10 mg. to 35 mg./24 hr.
   2nd trimester—rises from 35 mg. to 70 mg./24 hr.
   3rd trimester—rises from 70 mg. to 100 mg./24 hr., falling
      sharply before onset of labour and precipitately after
      delivery.
   Peak values are attained between 36th and 38th weeks.

Range in Normal Menstrual Cycle.—
   1. Follicular stage—0–0·1 mg./24 hr.
   2. 1–2 days after ovulation—3–5 mg./24 hr.
   3. Anovulatory cycle—0·75–1·5 mg./24 hr.

N.B.—**The amount is very variable, and estimation has no
clinical use.**

Range in Normal Males.—0–1 mg./24 hr.

Pathological.—
   Decrease in Output during Pregnancy.—
      1. Placental insufficiency.
      2. Toxæmia of pregnancy.
      3. Non-toxic accidental intra-uterine hæmorrhage.
      4. Fœtal death. If less than 5 mg./24 hr., then abortion is
         inevitable.

   Increased Output.—
      1. Chorionepithelioma. 8–15 mg./24 hr. has been reported.
      2. "Feminine" type of male pseudohermaphroditism. An
         excessive excretion of urine pregnanediol may be found.
      3. Stein-Leventhal syndrome (hyperthecosis ovarii). A
         marked increase in this condition has been found.
      4. Hypergonadism of adrenal origin.

N.B.—**The urine output of pregnanediol reflects placental
function. Its estimation may perhaps be used in the detection of
pregnancy.**

REFERENCES.—Coyle, M. G., Mitchell, F. L., Russell, C. S., and Paine,
    C. G. (1955), *J. Obstet. Gynæc. Brit. Emp.*, **2**, 291; Klopper, A., Michie,
    E. A., and Brown, J. B. (1955), *J. Endocrin.*, **12**, 209; Ober, W. B.,
    and Kaiser, G. A. (1961), *Amer. J. clin. Path.*, **35**, 297 (66 references).

PREGNANETRIOL IN URINE

Normal Output.—
1. Infants and children up to 6 years=0–0·2 mg./24 hr.
  Children 7–15 years=0·3–1·1 mg./24 hr.
2. Normal adults=0·1–3·0 mg./24 hr.

Pathological Increase.—
1. Congenital adrenal hyperplasia. Estimation is useful in both diagnosis and assessment of corticoid therapy.
2. Stein-Leventhal syndrome.

REFERENCE.—Prunty, F. T. G. (1961), *The Adrenal Cortex* (Ed. McGowan, G. K., and Sandler, M.), pp. 143–157. London: Pitman.

PROTEIN

SERUM PROTEINS.—
Normal Range.—
 Adult (serum)=6·3–7·8 g./100 ml.
 Newborn infant (plasma)=4·0–6·7 g./100 ml.
 Premature infant (plasma)=3·6–6·0 g./100 ml.
 It is worth noting that serum protein is increased temporarily by up to+10 per cent following vigorous exercise.

SERUM ALBUMIN.—
Normal Adult Range.—More than 3·0 g./100 ml.

Physiological.—Serum albumin half-life=17–26 days. Normal production in an adult=12 g./day. Of the normal body 300 g., 50 per cent is carried in the blood-stream and 50 per cent is in the extracellular space. The normal rate of albumin synthesis is near the maximum possible rate. In normal pregnancy the serum albumin falls progressively during the second and third trimesters, and remains low until about 3 months after delivery. This is due to an absolute increase in plasma volume, with associated increase in alpha-2 and beta-globulin fractions.

Pathological.—
 Decrease.—
  1. Decrease in rate of albumin synthesis.
  2. Increase in rate of degradation.
  3. Excessive loss of albumin.
  4. Any combination of (1), (2), and/or (3).
   a. After trauma or surgery (lowest values between fourth and tenth days).
   b. Bacterial endotoxin action.
   c. Myocardial infarction.
   d. Nephrotic syndrome.
   e. Rheumatoid arthritis.
   f. Burns.
   g. Liver disease.
   h. Malignancy.
   i. Chronic infection.
   j. Protein-losing gastroenteropathy, e.g., ulcerative colitis.
 I. *Hyperproteinæmia.—*
  1. *Normal or Reduced Albumin Concentration.—*
   a. *Gross Albumin Loss with Dehydration.—*
    i. Burns.

   ii. Ulcerative colitis.
   iii. Intestinal obstruction.
   iv. Generalized peritonitis.
   v. Chronic nephritis at the stage of polyuria.
   vi. Renal tubular damage, at the stage of recovery
       with gross diuresis.
   *b. Fluid Disturbance between Interstitial Fluid and
   Intravascular Fluid.*—
       Loss of extracellular fluid.
   c. Gross Increase in Globulin Fractions.—
       i. Portal cirrhosis.
       ii. Myeloma. Gross increase occurs in the abnormal
           protein fraction (alpha-, beta-, gamma-, M-protein
           type, or mixed type).
       iii. Sarcoidosis. (Some cases when active.)
       iv. Collagen diseases.
   *d. Dehydration associated with Conditions which may
   cause A/G Reversal.*—E.g., carcinomatosis.
2. *Normal Albumin Concentration.*—
   a. Simple Dehydration.—
       i. Inadequate fluid intake.
       ii. Excessive fluid loss:—
           α. Sweat.
           β. Vomit.
           γ. Gastric or small intestinal fluid aspiration.
           δ. Severe diarrhœa.
II. *Hypoproteinœmia.*—
   Low Albumin Concentration.—
   1. *Malnutrition.*—Low protein intake.
   2. *Loss of Albumin-rich Fluid.*—
       a. Nephrosis. Very large amounts of albumin may
           be lost in the urine.
       b. Intestinal loss, as in ulcerative colitis.
       c. Surface loss, e.g., burns.
   3. *Depressed Albumin Metabolism with Increased Globulin
       Formation.*—
       a. Uncomplicated liver disease:—
           i. Acute hepatitis.
           ii. Hepatic necrosis.
           iii. Cirrhosis, biliary or portal.
       b. Severe diabetic ketosis.
       c. Severe thyrotoxicosis (? rapid albumin turnover).
       d. Chronic nephritis (some cases).
       e. Untreated pernicious anæmia.
       f. Severe infections.
       g. Cachectic states.
       h. Scurvy.
   4. *Water Deviation.*—Increase in plasma volume without
       increase in total protein, i.e., gross œdema, ascites,
       effusions:—
       a. Congestive cardiac failure.
       b. Portal cirrhosis.
       c. Nephrosis.
       d. Peritonitis.
       e. Intestinal obstruction.

It has been found that in patients with "internal disorder":—

    i. Serum albumin >3 g. per cent—immediate mortality $=6$ per cent in 779 cases.

    ii. Serum albumin <3 g. per cent—immediate mortality $=33$ per cent in 779 cases.

Also patients with cirrhosis in whom serum albumin remains below 3·2 g. per cent despite treatment are unsuitable for portacaval or lienorenal anastomosis operation.

REFERENCES.—Hunt, A. H., and Lehmann, H. (1959), *Lancet*, **2**, 547; Wuhrmann, F. (1959), *Schweiz. med. Wschr.*, **89**, 343.

SERUM GLOBULIN.—

Normal Adult Range.—Up to 3·5 g./100 ml., depending on the method of estimation.

Although more information can be obtained from quantitative or qualitative opinion of changes in the various serum globulin fractions, the following very rough generalizations can be made:—

After excluding dehydration, fever, malnutrition, or laboratory error, it was found in 394 cases of hyperglobulinæmia:—

1. *Serum Globulin*: 3·9–4·2 g./100 ml.—
    a. 44·5 per cent of cases: diagnosis was not associated with the raised serum globulin level.
    b. 9·1 per cent of cases were either myeloma, sarcoidosis, or collagen disease.
    c. 17 per cent of cases: carcinoma.
    d. 20·6 per cent of cases: acute and chronic inflammation.
2. *Serum Globulin*: 4·21–4·99 g./100 ml.—
    a. 28 per cent of cases: diagnosis was not associated with the raised serum globulin level.
    b. 8·9 per cent of cases were either myeloma, sarcoidosis, or collagen disease.
    c. Commonest diagnoses in this group:—
        i. Liver disease (19·6 per cent).
        ii. Metastatic carcinoma (20·2 per cent).
        iii. Acute and chronic inflammation (22 per cent).
3. *Serum Globulin*: 5·0 g./100 ml. serum or more.—
    a. 8·4 per cent of cases: diagnosis was not associated with the raised serum globulin level.
    b. 43·3 per cent of cases: diagnosis was either myeloma, sarcoidosis, or collagen disease.
    c. 18·3 per cent of cases: diagnosis was liver disease.
    d. 20 per cent of cases: acute and chronic inflammation.

On paper electrophoretic separation, serum globulin separates into the following fractions:—

1. Alpha-1.
2. Alpha-2.
3. Beta.
4. Gamma.

These fractions can be further subdivided, but this is not considered here.

N.B.—It is important that minimum hæmostasis be used when blood is collected for serum protein estimation. Excessive stasis with congestion leads to changes in the hæmatocrit value, the total serum protein concentration, and the albumin/globulin ratio.

REFERENCE.—Feinstein, A. R., and Petersdorf, R. G. (1956), *Ann. intern. Med.*, **44**, 899.

SERUM ALPHA-GLOBULIN.—The alpha-globulin fractions carry alkaline phosphatase, complement endpiece, hypertensinogen, lipoproteins, pseudoglobulin, thyrotropin, mucoproteins, and C-reactive protein.

SERUM ALPHA-1 GLOBULIN.—

Normal Range.—1–5 per cent of total protein range 6·3–7·8 g./100 ml. serum.

Physiological.—Moderate increase occurs in the last six months of pregnancy.

Pathological.—
Increase.—
1. *Non-bacterial Tissue Damage.—*
    a. Slight increase follows coronary artery thrombosis and also bone fractures.
    b. Moderate increase follows X-ray irradiation.
2. *Acute Infections.*—There is a moderate increase in the early stages.
3. *Chronic Infections.*—There is a persistent slight increase.
4. *Collagen Diseases.*—Moderate increases in:—
    a. Systemic lupus erythematosus.
    b. Polyarteritis nodosa.
    c. Rheumatoid arthritis.
    d. Rheumatic fever in the early stages.
5. *Liver Disease.*—No consistent tendency to increase.
6. *Renal Diseases.*—Moderate increases in:—
    a. Acute nephritis.
    b. Chronic nephritis.
    c. Pyelonephritis.

Decrease.—
1. Hepatic necrosis.
2. Nephrosis.

SERUM ALPHA-2 GLOBULIN.—

Normal Range.—4·5–9·5 per cent of total serum protein range 6·3–7·8 g./100 ml.

Physiological.—The alpha-2 fraction is raised at birth, and falls progressively to normal during the subsequent 6 months.

In pregnancy the alpha-2 fraction increases moderately in the second trimester, and more markedly in the third trimester.

Pathological.—
Increase.—
1. *Non-infective Tissue Necrosis.*—Rapid increase occurs before the rise in the gamma fraction, in:—
    a. Coronary artery thrombosis.
    b. Bone fractures.
    c. X-ray irradiation.
2. *Acute Infection.*—Increase in the early stages.

3. *Chronic Infection.*—The increase persists. The level falls on recovery, before the gamma fraction falls.

4. *Collagen Diseases.*—
   a. Systemic lupus erythematosus. Marked increase.
   b. Polyarteritis nodosa. Marked increase.
   c. Rheumatoid arthritis. The level is raised, and does not fall with steroid therapy.
   d. Rheumatic fever. Increases occur in the acute phase (parallel with the serum C-reactive protein), and fall during quiescence or following steroid therapy.

5. *Liver Disease.*—
   a. Viral hepatitis. Slight to moderate increase (related to the increase in alpha-lipoprotein).
   b. Hepatic necrosis. If the necrosis is not too extensive there may be a slight increase.
   c. Cirrhosis. Moderate increases in both biliary and portal types.

6. *Renal Diseases.*—
   a. Acute nephritis. There is a moderate increase appearing in the early stages.
   b. Chronic nephritis. Moderate increase.
   c. Pyelonephritis. Moderate increase.
   d. Nephrosis. There is an increase with poor separation from the beta-globulin band.

7. *Malignancy.*—
   a. Myeloma. The alpha type shows a marked increase.
   b. Carcinoma. Moderate to marked increase.
   c. Lymphomas. There is a moderate increase.
   d. Hodgkin's disease (lymphadenoma). There is a moderate increase.

8. *Sarcoidosis.*—Frequently there is a marked increase. A moderate increase persists in quiescence.

9. *Cushing's Syndrome.*—There may be a slight to moderate increase.

FETOPROTEINS IN BLOOD.—Alpha-1 fetoprotein is a normal component of plasma at 6 weeks in the normal fœtus, with peak concentrations at 12–16 weeks. Normal synthesis of this protein ceases in the third trimester of pregnancy, and the protein is normally present in traces in the cord blood, but not detectable in infants after the first week of extra-uterine life.

Normal Range (at birth).—2·5–17 mg./100 ml.

Pathological.—
   Increase.—
   1. Primary carcinoma of the liver (hepatoma).
   2. Testicular teratoblastoma (in 10 per cent of cases).

REFERENCES.—Alpert, M. E., Uriel, J., and de Nechaud, B. (1968), *New Engl. J. Med.*, **278**, 984; Foli, A. K., Sherlock, S., and Adinolfi, M. (1969), *Lancet*, **2**, 1267; Editorial (1970), *Ibid.*, **1**, 397.

SERUM BETA-GLOBULIN.—

Normal Range.—11–16 per cent of total serum protein range 6·3–7·8 g./100 ml. The beta-globulin fraction carries lipoproteins, complement midpiece, fibrinolysin, isohæmagglutinins, luteinizing hormone, prothrombin, phospholipids, and cholesterol.

Physiological.—
1. Infants at birth may have a slightly raised beta fraction.
2. During the second trimester of normal pregnancy the beta fraction increases slightly. This increase becomes more marked in the final three months.

Pathological.—
Increase.—
1. *Liver Disease.—*
   a. Biliary cirrhosis. Marked increase.
   b. Viral hepatitis. Moderate increase in some cases. This is possibly caused by, or associated with, intra-hepatic biliary obstruction.
2. *Lipid Disorders.—*Marked increase in:—
   a. Primary xanthomatosis.
   b. Essential hyperlipæmia.
   c. Essential hypercholesterolæmia.
3. *Renal Diseases.—*Nephrosis. There is a marked increase with incomplete separation from the alpha-2 fraction.
4. *Myeloma.—*There is a marked increase in the beta-type.
5. *Polyarteritis Nodosa.—*There is a moderate increase in some cases.

Decrease.—
The beta fraction may be decreased in some cases of hepatic necrosis.

SERUM GAMMA-GLOBULIN.—
Normal Range (This includes the immunoglobulins).—

Age	Serum Gamma-globulin (mg./100 ml.)	Total Circulating Gamma-globulin (g.)
Birth	700–1000	1·4
4 weeks	250–650	0·9
8 weeks	200–400	0·7
12 weeks	250–400	0·8
24 weeks	270–600	1·25
1 year	450–700	2·5
3 years	600–900	4·0
Adult	750–1000	25·0

REFERENCE.—Martin, N. H. (1964), *Proc. Roy. Soc. Med.*, **57**, 752.

Normal Structure.—Gamma-globulins consist of three major classes of immunoglobulins. Each of these immunoglobulins consists of two pairs of polypeptide chains, a pair of "light" chains and a pair of "heavy" chains. The "light" chains, with a molecular weight of 20,000, may be κ or λ, and the "heavy" chains may be α or γ or μ, with a molecular weight of 60,000. The pair of "light" chains is coupled with the appropriate pair of "heavy" chains by disulphide linkages.

Immuno-globulin	Normal Chains	Age when Normal Adult Level reached
IgA	$\alpha_2\kappa_2$ or $\alpha_2\lambda_2$	15 years
IgG	$\gamma_2\kappa_2$ or $\gamma_2\lambda_2$	2 years
IgM	$\mu_2\kappa_2$ or $\mu_2\lambda_2$	6 months
IgD	$\delta_2\kappa_2$ or $\delta_2\lambda_2$	
IgE (IgND)		

Synonyms.—
IgA$=\beta_2$-A-globulin, γ_1-A-globulin, βX.
IgG$=$7-S-γ-globulin, γ-G-globulin, γ_2-globulin.
IgM$=$19-S-pentamer, β_2-M-globulin, γ_1M, 19-S-γ-globulin.

Immuno-globulin	*Molecular Weight*	*Serum Concentration*	*Half-life*
IgG	160,000	800–1500 mg./100 ml.	23 days
IgA	170,000 (monomer) 385,000 (dimer)	150–350 mg./100 ml.	5·8 days
IgM	900,000 (pentamer)	80–180 mg./100 ml.	5·1 days
IgD	180,000	1–5 mg./100 ml.	2·8 days
IgE (IgND)	200,000	0·0005 mg./100 ml.	2·3 days

In brief, IgG protects the body fluids, IgA protects the body surfaces, IgM protects the blood-stream, from foreign proteins. IgE mediates reaginic hypersensitivity.

Mean Normal Adult (MNA).—

IgA 248 mg./100 ml. 19 per cent
IgG 947 mg./100 ml. 73 per cent
IgM 94 mg./100 ml. 7 per cent
IgD 3 mg./100 ml.
} Normal pattern fluctuates by 20 per cent over a year.

In underdeveloped countries IgG and IgM occur in higher concentration than in Western Europe. IgA levels appear to be the same the world over. IgE is increased where worm infestation occurs.

Increase.—

Diffuse overproduction of immunoglobulins:—

1. Infection.
2. Sarcoidosis.
3. Beryllium poisoning.
4. Hyperimmunization.
5. Liver parenchymal diseases.
6. Reticulo-endothelial neoplasia.
7. Connective tissue (collagen) disorders.—
   a. Disseminated lupus erythematosus.
   b. Rheumatoid arthritis.
   c. Polyarteritis nodosa.
   d. Dermatomyositis.
8. Hypersensitivity diseases.—
   a. Serum sickness.
   b. Acquired auto-immune hæmolytic anæmia.
   c. Thyroiditis.

Overproduction of "monoclonal" immunoglobulins:—

1. Macroglobulinæmia (IgM).
2. Heavy-chain disease (?Fe fragment of IgG=result of deletion in end portion of heavy chain).
3. Lymphoma.
4. Unrelated neoplasm.
5. Idiopathic.
6. Myeloma.—
   a. IgG.
   b. IgA.
   c. IgD. Urine always contains Bence Jones protein. High incidence of intra-osseous tumours occurs in younger subjects. Paper electrophoresis—proteins migrate with β-band.

REFERENCE.—Fahey, J. L., Carbone, P. P., Rowe, D. S., and Bachman, R. (1968), *Amer. J. Med.*, 45, 373.

d. IgE. Plasma-cell leukæmia in peripheral blood. No punched-out holes in bones on X-ray.

REFERENCES.—Johansson, S. G. O. (1967), *Lancet*, 2, 951; Editorial (1969), *New Engl. J. Med.*, 281, 502.

Decrease.—
  Diminished production of immunoglobulins:—
    Type I IgA↓, IgM↓, IgG normal.
    Type II IgA↓, IgG↓, IgM↑.
    Type III IgG↓.
    Type IV IgA↓.
    Type V IgM↓.
    Type VI Apparently normal levels of IgG, IgA, IgM.
    Type VII IgG↓, IgM↓, IgA↑.
      (Types IV and V are far more frequently found than the other types.)

REFERENCES.—Hobbs, J. R. (1968), *Lancet*, 1, 110; Waldmann, T. A (1969), *New Engl. J. Med.*, 281, 1170.

SERUM GLYCOPROTEINS.—Glycoproteins consist of proteins linked to carbohydrates by covalent bonds, characteristically containing two or more of the following:—
  D-Galactose, D-mannose, D-glucose, L-fucose, D-xylose, N-acetyl-D-glucosamine, N-acetyl-D-galactosamine, and various derivatives of neuraminic acid. The carbohydrate content ranges from 1 to 80 per cent of the weight of the molecule, and the molecular weight ranges from 14,500 to 1,000,000.
  These very important substances include:—

Haptoglobin	Chorionic
Transferrin	gonadotrophin
Immunoglobulins	Fibrinogen
Thyroglobulin	Prothrombin
Skin collagen	Alpha-glycoprotein
Cell-membrane glycoprotein	Cæruloplasmin
Connective-tissue glycoprotein	
Basement-membrane glycoprotein.	

Non-specific glycoproteins increase in the plasma in many inflammatory conditions.
  In primary hepatoma fetuin appears in the plasma.

REFERENCE.—Spiro, R. G. (1969), *New Engl. J. Med.*, 281, 991, 1043.

PLASMA HAPTOGLOBINS.—
Normal Range.—28–190 mg./100 ml. Haptoglobins, of which four are known, are mucoproteins normally present singly or in different combinations in the alpha-2 fraction of the plasma globulins. Small amounts of hæmoglobin liberated intravascularly are firmly bound to these substances, and eventually metabolized and eliminated via the reticulo-endothelial system. Up to 135 mg./100 of plasma can be bound in this way. When this level is exceeded, hæmoglobin is carried by beta-globulin and albumin, and appears in the urine.
  Haptoglobins are normally not demonstrable in cord blood. A small percentage of the normal population have no demonstrable haptoglobins.

Pathological.—

Increase.—

1. Acute inflammation.
2. Neoplastic infiltration and destruction of tissue.
3. Degeneration of body tissues.

Decrease.—

1. Intravascular hæmolysis, e.g.:—

   a. Paroxysmal nocturnal hæmoglobinuria.

   b. March hæmoglobinuria.

   The plasma level of haptoglobin appears to be related inversely to the activity of the hæmolytic process. In remission, the haptoglobin level is normal. On the other hand, when hæmolysis is severe enough to produce an apparent red-cell life of 17 days (normal = 120 days) then plasma haptoglobin is absent. Possibly there is an excessively slow rate of formation or liberation of haptoglobin, or far more probably persistent hæmolysis uses up all available haptoglobin. The haptoglobin–hæmoglobin complex is lost from the circulation at the rate of 13 mg./100 ml./hr.

2. Pernicious anæmia ⎫ Probably due at least partly
3. Hepatocellular failure ⎬ to impaired formation.

References.—Aber, G. M., Neale, F. C., and Northam, B. E. (1957), *Brit. med. J.*, **2**, 1368; Allison, A. C., and Ap Rees, W. (1957), *Ibid.*, **2**, 1137; Laurell, C. B., and Nyman, M. (1957), *Blood*, **12**, 493; Nosslin, B. F., and Nyman, M. (1958), *Lancet*, **1**, 1000.

SERUM LIPOPROTEINS.—Because of great instability it is important that only fresh, fasting and unfrozen sera be examined by electrophoresis. The various fractions can be separated.—

1. Chylomicrons. High percentage of triglycerides and low protein content.
2. Pre-β liproproteins. Containing more cholesterol and phospholipids, but still over 50 per cent triglycerides.
3. β-Lipoproteins, 50 per cent cholesterol, 10 per cent triglyceride, 20 per cent protein.
4. α-Lipoproteins (high density), 45 per cent protein, 26 per cent lipoprotein.

Pathological.—

Increase.—

Hyperlipidæmias.—

1. Type I (rare). Gross increase in plasma neutral fat, moderate increase in cholesterol and phospholipids. Chylomicrons+++.
2. Type II. Plasma neutral fat not increased. Cholesterol and phospholipids increased.
3. Type III. Increases in both pre-β and β-lipoproteins, with turbid serum, increased triglycerides and cholesterol.
4. Type IV. Increase in pre-β-lipoprotein with increased triglycerides and cholesterol. Turbid serum.
5. Type V. Increase in pre-β-lipoprotein and chylomicrons.

Turbid serum. Increased triglycerides with normal or slightly increased cholesterol.

REFERENCES.—Fredrickson, D. S., Levy, R. I., and Lees, R. (1967), *New Engl. J. Med.*, **276**, 34, 94, 148, 215, and 273; Strisower, E. H., Adamson, G., and Strisower, B. (1968), *Amer. J. Med.*, **45**, 488.

Decrease.—

1. A-β-lipoproteinæmia. Familial absence or gross reduction in β-lipoprotein.
2. A-α-lipoproteinæmia. Familial absence or gross reduction in α-lipoprotein (Tangier disease).

REFERENCE.—Lane, R. F. (1969), *J. Med. Lab. Technol.*, **26**, 212.

SERUM MUCOPROTEINS.—

Normal Range.—Normally about 1–2 per cent of total serum protein is present in the form of mucoprotein.

1. Adult males—138 $\pm$ 5·62 mg./100 ml.
2. Adult females—134·3 $\pm$ 5·58 mg./100 ml.

Definition.—A mucoprotein is a substance in which protein and mucopolysaccharide radicals are linked in firm chemical union, the former being the major constituent to the extent of 70–90 per cent and the latter containing more than 4 per cent of hexosamine by arbitrary definition.

Pathological.—
Increase.—

1. Carcinoma.
2. Collagen diseases.
3. Infections.
4. Trauma, e.g., surgical operation.

Decrease.—

1. Some endocrine conditions in the absence of infection or inflammation.
2. Liver diseases, in the absence of infection, inflammation, or cell regeneration.
3. Low serum mucoprotein levels have been found in some cases of myeloma.
4. ACTH or adrenal corticoid therapy.

*N.B.—***At present, the wide spread of values found in any one clinical condition suggests that it is not a useful routine investigation.**

URINE MUCOPROTEINS.—The urine excretion is proportional to the serum concentration. Some of the urine mucoprotein is in fact haptoglobin.

1. Normal adult males—156 $\pm$ 6·7 mg./24 hr.
2. Normal adult females—111 $\pm$ 6·15 mg./24 hr.

*N.B.—***Further research is needed before the clinical value of this estimation can be decided.**

REFERENCE.—Lockey, E., Anderson, A. J., and Maclagan, N. F. (1956), *Brit. J. Cancer*, **10**, 209.

SERUM PYROGLOBULINS.—Serum pyroglobulins may be defined as globulins which gel at 45–55° C., and which may not re-dissolve on cooling. Their significance is not known, apart from the fact that they have been detected in myelomatosis.

PARAPROTEINÆMIA.—Paraproteinæmia may be defined as a condition in which serum globulins normally absent, or present in only minimal quantities, are found in greatly increased amounts:—

1. *Myeloma Globulins.*—
   a. Alpha type. Uncommon type.
   b. Beta type. Uncommon type.
   c. Gamma type. Common type.
   d. "M" type (peak between beta and gamma fractions).
   e. Mixed type (peaks in both beta and gamma fractions).

2. *Cryoglobulins.*—A cryoglobulin may be defined as a globulin present in serum or plasma collected and separated at 37° C., which gels at 4° C. (although some specimens gel at temperatures above 4° C. and below 35° C.). The gel re-dissolves as the temperature rises towards 37° C.

   On paper electrophoresis, the protein involved often has the mobility of a gamma-globulin, but it may move with the slow beta fraction.

   The protein may be found in sera from cases of:—
   a. Myeloma with/without Raynaud's phenomenon.
   b. Chronic nephritis.
   c. Reticuloses.
   d. Chronic lymphatic leukæmia.
   e. Periarteritis nodosa.
   f. Some cases of Raynaud's syndrome, cause not known.
   g. Rheumatoid arthritis.
   h. Cirrhosis of the liver.
   i. Kala-azar.
   j. Subacute bacterial endocarditis.
   k. Macroglobulinæmia.
   l. "Essential" cryoglobulinæmia (3 cases described).
   m. Rarely, in:—
      i. Coronary disease.
      ii. Asthma.
      iii. Urticaria.
      iv. Brucellosis.
      v. Gout.
      vi. Malaria.

3. *Macroglobulins.*—Macroglobulins may be defined as globulins with a molecular weight of approximately 1,600,000. Separation with the Svedborg ultracentrifuge gives an S_f value of more than 18 (values of up to 25 S_f units have been found). On paper electrophoresis the protein lies near the beta-1 globulin fraction between the beta and gamma bands. It is best demonstrated in either agar-agar or starch gel electrophoresis.

   The serum relative viscosity ratio is increased:—

$$\frac{\text{Serum viscosity at } 13° \text{ C.}}{\text{Serum viscosity at } 37° \text{ C.}} = \text{More than } 120$$

Serum containing macroglobulin may exhibit gel formation similar to the action of cryoglobulins. It is possible that the particular macroglobulin molecule does not contain hydroxyproline.

As with cryoglobulins, intravascular precipitation of the protein may cause purpura.

The presence of the protein may be demonstrated by water dilution. One drop of serum added to distilled water results in turbidity, which disappears in sodium chloride solution. This test is not specific.

The one-stage prothrombin estimation may be prolonged due to antagonism to the action of Factors V and VII.

Cryoglobulin may also be present. Also Bence Jones protein may be present in the urine.

Macroglobulinæmia may be:—

    a. Primary.
    b. Secondary:—
        i. Nephrosis.
        ii. Lupus erythematosus.

REFERENCES.—Waldenström, J. (1952), *Advanc. internal Med.*, **5**, 398; Editorial (1956), *Brit. med. J.*, **1**, 1475; Editorial (1956), *Ibid.*, **2**, 409; Mackay, I. R., Taft, L. I., and Woods, E. F. (1957), *Ibid.*, **1**, 561.

C-REACTIVE PROTEIN (ACUTE PHASE PROTEIN) IN SERUM.

—Serum C-reactive protein (associated with the alpha-globulin fraction) is not normally detectable in serum. Following any acute inflammatory change and before any rise in the erythrocyte sedimentation rate, C-reactive protein appears in the serum. On recovery, the C-reactive protein disappears before the erythrocyte sedimentation rate falls to normal. For example, C-reactive protein appears in the serum within 24 hours of myocardial infarction, and begins to diminish by the third day.

C-reactive protein disappears when the inflammatory condition is suppressed by either steroid or salicylate therapy.

Steroids and salicylates do not act on the C-reactive protein directly.

REFERENCES.—Anderson, H. C., and McCarty, M. (1950), *Amer. J. Med.*, **8**, 445; Yocum, R. S., and Doerner, A. A. (1957), *Arch. intern. Med.*, **99**, 74; Eastham, R. D., Szekely, P., and Davison, K. (1958), *Ann. rheum. Dis.*, **17**, 314, 319.

PROTEIN-BOUND POLYSACCHARIDES IN SERUM.—

These substances include:—

1. Glucosamine.
2. Non-glucose hexosamine. (Galactose : mannite: : 1·0 : 1·0.)
3. Fucose.
4. Sialic acid.

Any increase in protein-bound polysaccharides is generally paralleled by increases in the serum protein fractions which carry the polysaccharides. In abnormal conditions the composition of the various serum protein fractions are not changed; only their relative and absolute amounts change (cf. paraproteinæmia). After paper electrophoresis of serum it is possible to demonstrate changes in the glycoprotein fractions in disease (Goa, 1955).

1. *Serum Glucosamine Polysaccharide.*—
    a. Normal children—52–69 mg./100 ml.
    b. Normal adults—61–78 mg./100 ml.
       The normal level rises with age.

2. *Serum Non-glucosamine Hexosamine.*—
    a. Normal children (3–8 years)—94–118 mg./100 ml.
    b. Normal adults—93–126 mg./100 ml.
       The normal level rises with age.

Both glucosamine and non-glucosamine hexosamine are normal components of serum mucoprotein, and also of various other serum protein fractions. Their concentrations are increased in active infections, collagen diseases (including rheumatoid arthritis), carcinoma, lymphadenoma, macro-globulinæmia, and in about 50 per cent of cases of diabetes mellitus. The levels decrease towards normal on recovery. Their estimation has been used in the assessment of activity in cases of rheumatic fever in children.

REFERENCES.—Shetlar, M. R., Foster, J. V., Kelly, K. H., and Everett, M. R. (1948), *Proc. Soc. exp. Biol., N.Y.*, **67**, 125; (1948), *Ibid.*, **69**, 507; Kelley, V. C. (1952), *J. Pediat.*, **40**, 405, 413; Goa, J. (1955), *Scand. J. clin. Lab. Invest.*, **7**, Suppl. 22; Weiden, S. (1958), *J. clin. Path.*, **11**, 177.

PROTEIN IN URINE.—
Normal Output.—
1. Up to 71 mg./24 hr.
2. Normal A/G ratio = 0·65.

It is probable that the normal glomerular filtrate contains some protein. This protein is almost completely reabsorbed by the renal tubular cells.

PROTEINURIA.—
1. *Functional.*—
    a. After severe exercise.
    b. Essential orthostatic proteinuria.
    c. Pregnancy.
    d. In some women in the pre-menstrual phase.
2. *Organic.*—
    a. *Pre-renal.*—
        i. Congestive cardiac failure.
        ii. Tumours pressing on the renal vein.
        iii. Partial thrombosis of the renal vein.
        iv. Severe anæmia.
        v. Severe shock.
        vi. Some cases of liver disease.
        vii. Febrile conditions.
        viii. After convulsions.
    b. *Renal.*—
        i. Nephritis. Acute and chronic phases.
        ii. Nephrosis.
        iii. Eclampsia.
        iv. Pyelonephritis.
        v. Pyelitis.
        vi. Drugs and poisons, e.g., mercuric chloride.

vii. Surgical operation (maximal on third and fourth days).

c. *Post-renal.*—Diseases of ureters, bladder, prostate, or urethra. (*See also* BENCE JONES PROTEIN IN URINE.)

REFERENCE.—McGarry, E., Sehon, A. H., and Rose, B. (1955), *J. clin. Invest.*, 34, 832.

PROTEIN IN CEREBROSPINAL FLUID.—
Normal Range.—
1. Ventricular fluid—Less than 15 mg./100 ml.
2. Cisternal fluid—Less than 25 mg./100 ml.
3. Lumbar fluid—Normal men—less than 60 mg./100 ml. Normal women—less than 50 mg./100 ml.
4. During the first year of life the normal range for the lumbar fluid may extend up to 80 mg./100 ml.
5. The normal adult albumin/globulin ratio is 2 : 1. During the first year of life this ratio is 1 : 1.
6. The cerebrospinal fluid contains some pre-albumin, and the globulin present is mainly gamma-globulin.

Pathological.—
Increase.—
   (Elevated cerebrospinal fluid protein is due to increased vascular permeability to albumin, not due to delay in removal of protein from the CSF. The normal CSF albumin turnover rate=17·3 mg./100 ml./day.)
1. *Acute Infection* (*Meningitis*). (Both albumin and globulin increase.)—
   a. Bacteria (e.g., *Meningococci*).
   b. Spirochætes (e.g., *T. pallida*).
   c. Rickettsia.
   d. Viruses.
   e. Fungi.
2. *Chronic Inflammation.—*
   a. General paralysis of the insane. A high cell-count indicates active disease which improves with treatment; a low cell-count indicates a static process which does not improve much with treatment.
   b. Disseminated sclerosis.
   c. Tuberculosis.
3. *Intrathecal Therapy.—*
   a. Streptomycin.
   b. Tuberculin.
4. *Intracranial Tumours.*—Especially acoustic neuroma. The finding of a higher protein concentration in one ventricle may help in the detection and localization of a tumour. Not all tumours show an increase in cerebrospinal fluid protein.
5. *Subarachnoid Hæmorrhage.*—Plasma proteins enter the cerebrospinal fluid.

N.B.—**A fibrin clot may develop if the protein level exceeds 200 mg./100 ml. (i.e., there is sufficient fibrinogen).**

6. *Cerebral Abscess.*—The protein concentration in the cerebrospinal fluid is raised, particularly if the abscess is near to the surface.

7. *Block.*—Below a block, serum albumin diffuses into the stagnant fluid, and the protein concentration rises. The fluid becomes progressively more pigmented (yellow—Froin's syndrome).

8. *Acute Polyneuritis.*—The cell-count does not rise in parallel with the protein increase in:—
   a. Diabetes mellitus.
   b. Diphtheritic polyneuritis.
   c. Landry's paralysis.
   d. Guillain-Barré syndrome.
   e. Wernicke's encephalopathy.

9. *Myxœdema.*—The mechanism for the increased cerebrospinal fluid protein concentration is not known. The level may reach 200 mg./100 ml.

10. *Lead Encephalitis.*—Especially in young children. But lumbar puncture in these cases can be very dangerous because of medullary herniation. Decompression with intravenous urea beforehand may be useful.

11. *Subacute Combined Degeneration of the Cord.*—Moderate increases up to 100 mg./100 ml. occur.

Specimens taken after air encephalography have lower protein concentrations than before air encephalography. The first specimen should be tested.

N.B.—**It is important to check the normal range of the laboratory. Many different methods of estimation are used.**

REFERENCES.—Yeoman, W. B. (1955), *J. clin. Path.*, **8**, 252; Cutler, R. W. P., Deuel, R. K., and Barlow, C. F. (1967), *Arch. Neurol.*, **17**, 261; Hunter, R., Jones, M., and Malleson, A. (1969), *J. Neurol. Sci.*, **9**, 11.

IMMUNOGLOBULINS IN CEREBROSPINAL FLUID.—

a. IgG.—
   Normal Results.—1·44 ± 0·53 mg. per cent.
   Pathological Increase.—
   1. Multiple sclerosis.
   2. Post-vaccinial encephalitis.
   3. Measles encephalitis.
   4. Neurosyphilis.
   5. Meningitis.
   6. Obstruction of spinal canal.
   7. Systemic lupus erythematosus.

   Decrease.—Epilepsy.
   (Normal results have been found in degenerative brain lesions, myeloneuropathy. No constant pattern of results has been found with brain tumours.)

b. IgA and IgM are only found in the CSF when the CSF protein content is abnormally raised. IgM is increased in trypanosomiasis.

REFERENCES.—Cutler, R. W. P., Walters, G. V., Hammerstad, J. P., and Merler, E. (1967), *Arch. Neurol.*, **17**, 620; Takase, S., and Yoshida, M. (1969), *Tohoku J. exp. Med.*, **98**, 189; Riddoch, D., and Thompson, R. A. (1970), *Lancet*, **1**, 396.

PROTEIN DIGESTION TEST.—1·3 g. gelatin/kg. body-weight

is given orally in 200 ml. of flavoured water after overnight fast. Blood samples are collected at 0, 1, and 3 hours.

Normal Results.—The blood amino-acid level rises by more than 3–4 mg./100 ml. in one hour, continuing to rise by more than 7–8 mg./100 ml. in three hours.

Pathological.—

1. *Cystic Fibrosis of the Pancreas.*—The blood amino-acid level fails to rise by more than 2·5 mg./100 ml.
2. This test has also been used in adults in an attempt to detect chronic pancreatitis, but the test is only positive in the presence of gross pancreatic damage.

   The author found that gelatin samples vary, and that the rate of absorption in apparently normal adults varies widely. Thus, the test is best confined to children.

REFERENCE.—West, C. D., Wilson, J. L., and Eyles, R. (1946), *Amer. J. Dis. Child.*, 72, 251.

PSEUDOCHOLINESTERASE AND RED CELL CHOLINESTERASE. *See* Cholinesterase, p. 43

PYROGEN TEST OF HYPOTHALAMIC-PITUITARY-ADRENAL FUNCTION

After injection of a pyrogen material, plasma cortisol estimations are made. In normal subjects the minimum rise in plasma cortisol is +8 μg./100 ml. Growth hormone concentrations are variable after pyrogen, and no consistent response has been found in normal subjects. Probably the insulin-induced hypoglycæmic response is a more sensitive method for detecting minor changes in the hypothalamic-pituitary-adrenal axis.

REFERENCES.—Kimball, H. R., Lipsett, M. B., Odell, W. D., and Wolff, S. M. (1968), *J. clin. Endocr. Metab.*, 28, 337; Carroll, B. J., Pearson, Margaret J., and Martin, F. R. (1969), *Metabolism*, 18, 476; Jacobs, H. S., and Nabarro, J. D. N. (1969), *Quart. J. Med.*, 38, 475.

PYRUVIC ACID

PYRUVIC ACID IN BLOOD.—
Normal Range.—0·5–1·0 mg./100 ml.

$$\left(\frac{\text{mg./litre}}{88} = \text{mmol./litre.} \right)$$

Vitamin B_1 (thiamine), when phosphorylated, acts as a co-carboxylase:—

$$\text{Pyruvate} \begin{cases} \text{acetate} \\ CO_2 \end{cases}$$

Physiological.—

1. *Glucose Ingestion.*—After glucose ingestion the blood pyruvate rises. In diabetes mellitus this rise does not occur until insulin has also been given.
2. *Strenuous Exercise.*—This is followed by a rapid rise in blood pyruvate within one hour, with subsequent rapid fall.

Pathological.—
Increase.—

1. Acute advanced beri-beri (vitamin-B_1 deficiency). Many cases of alcoholic polyneuritis are due to vitamin-B_1 deficiency.

2. Very advanced liver disease.
3. Severe cardiac failure (i.e., exertion involving accessory respiratory muscles in the presence of anoxæmia).
4. Uræmia. It is possible that accumulated toxic products act as a block.
5. Some acute infections. Presumably due to anoxæmia and excessive carbohydrate metabolism.
6. Metal poisons. The following metals inhibit pyruvate oxidation:—
   a. Arsenic.
   b. Antimony.
   c. Gold.
   d. Mercury.
7. *Argemone mexicale* (an alkaloid contaminating some mustard-seed cooking-oil samples) inhibits pyruvate oxidation.
8. Bracken and "horses' tails" both contain a specific thiaminase. They can cause "staggers" in sheep and horses.
9. Raised levels have been reported in some cases of multiple sclerosis. The cause for this has not been discovered.
10. Raised levels have been reported in unstable diabetes mellitus (insulin sensitive), with normal levels in stable diabetes (insulin resistant).
11. Elevation of blood pyruvate can be demonstrated in cases of diabetic ketosis (after removal of aceto-acetic acid).
12. Hepatolenticular degeneration. Reverts to normal after treatment with copper-chelating agent.

N.B.—**It is important that blood is taken only from patients who are fasting and at rest. A cooled syringe and iced reagents must be used.**

McArdle's Syndrome: Blood lactate and pyruvate do not rise after exercise.

Unless special care is taken, false high readings may be obtained, or pyruvate may be lost from the blood sample soon after collection.

REFERENCES.—Friedmann, T. E., and Haugen, G. E. (1943), *J. biol. Chem.*, **147**, 415; (1945), *Ibid.*, **157**, 673; Hill, L., and Walshe, J. M. (1959), *Lancet*, **2**, 444; Walton, J. N. (1964), *Ibid.*, **1**, 447.

PYRUVATE METABOLISM TEST.—

Method.—With the fasting patient at rest in bed, a fasting blood sample is taken for pyruvate estimation. Two doses of 50 g. of glucose each in 200 ml. of water are given at 0 and 30 minutes after the fasting blood sample.

Blood samples are then taken at 60 and 90 minutes.

Results.—

Fasting Blood Level.—Between 0·5 and 1·0 mg./100 ml. (Average = 0·76 mg./100 ml.)

60-minute Specimen.—Average level = 0·92 mg./100 ml.

90-minute Specimen.—Average level = 0·94 mg./100 ml.

Pathological.—

1. *Normal Fasting Pyruvate, but Excessive Prolonged Rise after Glucose Ingestion* (i.e., > 1·4 mg./100 ml.):—

   a. *Responding to Vitamin-B₁ Therapy.—*
      i. Subacute and chronic moderate vitamin-B₁ deficiency.
      ii. Moderate congestive cardiac failure.
      iii. Obese, insulin resistant, diabetics on insulin.

   b. *Not Responding to Vitamin-B₁ Therapy.—*
      i. Where polyneuritis is due to blocking of pyruvate metabolism (e.g., heavy metals), the curve is abnormally raised and prolonged. Vitamin B₁ produces no improvement.
         (Where polyneuritis is due to other factors, the curve is usually normal.)
      ii. Pernicious anæmia with subacute combined degeneration of the spinal cord. The abnormal pyruvate curve falls back to normal after vitamin-B₁₂ therapy.
      iii. Hepatolenticular degeneration (untreated). Reverts to normal after treatment with copper-chelating agents.

2. *Normal Fasting Pyruvate with No Rise after Oral or Intravenous Glucose.—*

   a. Untreated diabetes mellitus.
   b. Thin, insulin deficient, diabetic treated with insulin.
   Injection of 10 g. sodium pyruvate intravenously has shown a slower decay rate than normal in diabetics, which is not corrected by insulin or oral hypoglycæmic agents.

REFERENCES.—Joiner, C. L., McArdle, B., and Thompson, R. H. S. (1950), *Brain*, **73**, 431; Lawrence, R. D. (1951), *Brit. med. J.*, **1**, 373; King, E. J. (1956), *Micro-analysis in Medical Biochemistry*, 3rd ed., pp. 217, 218. London: Churchill; Smith, M. J. H., and Taylor, K. W. (1956), *Brit. med. J.*, **2**, 1035; Moorhouse, J. A. (1964), *Lancet*, **1**, 689.

RENIN IN PLASMA

A method is available.

REFERENCE.—Haas, E., Gould, A. B., and Goldblatt, H. (1968), *Lancet*, **1**, 657.

SALICYLATE IN PLASMA

Therapeutic plasma salicylate levels of 20–40 mg./100 ml. have been recommended. At levels of about 40 mg./100 ml. tinnitus develops. In salicylate poisoning the blood concentration may exceed 100 mg./100 ml.

A very rapid accurate method is available, which does not require any extraction. In addition, by heating the serum-reagent mixture in a boiling water bath for 10 minutes, and subsequently cooling the mixture to room temperature before reading the result, the effect of associated ketone bodies can be eliminated. This may be important when diabetes mellitus is also present.

REFERENCE.—Trinder, P. (1954), *Biochem. J.*, **57**, 301.

SALT DEPRIVATION TEST.—

With safer and more accurate tests of adrenal function available, this test should be discontinued.

REFERENCE.—Cutler, H. H., Power, M. H., and Wilder, R. M. (1938), *J. Amer. med. Ass.*, **111**, 117.

SALIVA ELECTROLYTES

SODIUM, POTASSIUM, AND CHLORIDE.—
Normal Range.—
1. Sodium—26·4 ± 11·8 mEq./litre, varying greatly with flow rate.
2. Potassium—19·7 ± 3·9 mEq./litre, unaffected by flow rate.
3. Chloride—29·0 ± 8·8 mEq./litre, varying slightly with flow rate.

After DOCA the sodium and chloride concentrations fall, and the potassium concentration rises. This also occurs in congestive cardiac failure and adrenocortical hyperactivity.

The sodium/potassium ratio falls in Cushing's syndrome. Unfortunately the saliva electrolyte range is wide, and the different responses to various stimuli make the estimations of doubtful use. This is especially so, since it is difficult to obtain a discrete specimen of saliva.

REFERENCE.—White, A. G., Entmacher, P. S., Rubin, G., and Leiter, L. (1955), *J. clin. Invest.*, **34**, 246.

SODIUM

SODIUM IN CEREBROSPINAL FLUID.—This estimation is of no clinical importance. The concentration in the cerebrospinal fluid is approximately the same as in the plasma.

SODIUM IN FÆCES.—The normal daily excretion of sodium in the stools is < 10 mEq. This may increase to more than 60 mEq./day in severe diarrhœa.

Although fæcal sodium estimations are only performed in metabolic balance studies, this potential site of sodium loss should be remembered.

SODIUM IN GASTRIC JUICE.—
Normal Concentration.—
1. Non-parietal juice—160 mEq./litre (mmol./litre).
2. Parietal juice—<10 mEq./litre (mmol./litre).

SODIUM IN PLASMA.—
Normal Range.—
  Males.—
    Mean—139·3 mEq./litre (mmol./litre).
    Range—135–143 mEq./litre (mmol./litre).
  Females.—
    Mean—139·1 mEq./litre (mmol./litre).
    Range—135–143 mEq./litre (mmol./litre).

REFERENCE.—Flynn, F. V. (1969), *Ann. Clin. Biochem.*, **6**, 1.

By variations in the rate of renal excretion of sodium and in the volume of the extracellular fluid, the normal range of plasma sodium concentration is maintained as long as possible in the presence of sodium excess or deficiency. The finding of a normal plasma sodium concentration does not necessarily indicate a normal body sodium balance, nor does it exclude total body sodium excess or deficiency.

It is essential to assess clinically:—
1. The state of hydration of the tissues.
2. The intake and output of fluids and electrolytes during the previous days.
3. The presence or absence of associated deficiency or excess of body potassium.

N.B.—In the presence of sodium deficiency with adequate body potassium, potassium derived from the intracellular fluid is excreted in the urine in place of sodium (some of which enters the cells with hydrogen ions). Thus, potassium from the intracellular fluid "spares" the extracellular sodium, and hence the extracellular fluid.

Pathological.—
Increase.—
1. *Dehydration.*—Following rigid restriction of water intake, or excessive sweating with poor water intake, the extracellular fluid volume progressively shrinks, the plasma sodium concentration being maintained within the normal range. After 36–48 hours (after 24–36 hours in a young child) the plasma sodium level increases, when the volume of fluid available is less than that required to eliminate the excess electrolytes and waste products.
2. *Excess Saline Therapy.*—Normally the kidneys can rapidly eliminate excess salt, but when cases of diabetic ketosis are treated with saline and insulin, the plasma sodium concentration may rise until normal renal function has been restored. Similarly, the kidneys of young children cannot cope with the excess salt when "normal" saline is transfused.
3. *Head Injury.*—Following head injury, the plasma sodium may rise above the normal range. This may be associated with dehydration due to poor fluid intake, but may also be secondary to hypothalamic damage or irritation.
4. *Steroid Therapy.*—Excessive DOCA and adrenal cortical hormone therapy lead to water retention with marked renal tubular sodium reabsorption.

Decrease (plasma sodium only falls after a 70-kg. man has lost 350–500 mEq. of sodium).—

Plasma sodium <120 mEq./litre results in weakness.
Plasma sodium <110 mEq./litre results in bulbar or pseudo-bulbar palsy.
Plasma sodium 90–105 mEq./litre results in severe neurological signs and symptoms.

1. *Gastro-intestinal Loss.—*
   a. Vomiting and continuous gastric aspiration, resulting in relative depletion of chloride and hydrogen ions (developing metabolic alkalosis), can lead to an increase in plasma sodium concentration in the presence of gross dehydration.
   Continuous gastric aspiration for 4–5 days can remove 93 g. of chloride as sodium chloride (i.e., more than half the total body chloride).

    b. Small intestinal aspiration or fistula. The loss of sodium per day (430 mEq.) is greater than the loss of chloride (270 mEq.).

    c. Diarrhœa. 60 mEq. of sodium and 60 mEq. of chloride may be lost per day during diarrhœa. Where the stools are similar to ileal fluid, the losses are far greater. Thus 600 mEq. of sodium and 550 mEq. of chloride may be lost each day from an ileostomy.

    d. Salt-removing resin added to the diet, or a low sodium chloride intake, or both, will reduce the plasma sodium level.

2. *Sweating,* with adequate water intake, and inadequate salt replacement, especially if sweating is profuse.

3. *Renal Loss.—*

    a. Obligatory loss. In diabetic ketosis the high concentration of glucose in the urine produces a diuresis, and the organic acids are excreted, combined with sodium and potassium. The normal buffering mechanisms of the kidneys are depressed, enhancing this loss of sodium and potassium.

    b. Tubular damage. In the late stages of renal disease the renal tubules cease to reabsorb sodium satisfactorily.

    Mercurial diuretics inhibit reabsorption of sodium by the renal tubules.

    Steroid deficiency in Addison's disease results in impaired sodium reabsorption by the renal tubules. This also occurs in adrenal failure secondary to hypopituitarism.

4. *Paracentesis.—*Much sodium can be lost when large volumes of ascitic fluid are regularly removed. In addition, these cases are often on restricted sodium chloride intake.

5. *Expansion of Extracellular Fluid.—*

    a. Water intoxication, e.g., after excess parenteral fluid.

    b. Hypothermia. Glucose solution acts as a relatively inert extracellular fluid volume expander when the body temperature is lowered.

    c. Lobar pneumonia and other infections.

6. *Carcinoma.—*Hyponatræmia develops in some cases of carcinoma probably as a result of:—

    a. Excessive production of antidiuretic hormone.

    b. Reduced production of aldosterone.

    c. Renal tubular lesion.

7. Hyponatræmia may develop in:—

    a. Acute intermittent porphyria.

    b. Variegate porphyria.

References.—Rosenheim, M. L. (1951), *Lancet,* **2**, 505; Wynn, V., and Rob, C. G. (1954), *Ibid.,* **1**, 587; Clarke, E., Evans, B. M., MacIntyre, I., and Milne, M. D. (1955), *Clin. Sci.,* **14**, 421; Editorial (1964), *Lancet,* **1**, 317.

SODIUM, CHLORIDE, AND POTASSIUM IN SWEAT.—

Normal.—

    Sodium—10–80 mEq./litre.

    Chloride—4–60 mEq./litre.

The sodium concentration rises as the rate of flow increases, i.e., reabsorption of sodium by the sweat-gland cells is "swamped".

Potassium is secreted at a higher concentration in sweat than in plasma. The ratio:—

$$\frac{\text{Sweat potassium}}{\text{Plasma potassium}} = 2 \cdot 2 \pm 0 \cdot 48.$$

Pathological.—

Increased Sodium and Chloride Secretion.—In cystic fibrosis of the pancreas (mucoviscidosis) during high rates of sweating:—

1. Sodium—80–190 mEq./litre.
2. Chloride—50–160 mEq./litre.

This abnormally high rate is unaffected by salt restriction, hot weather (many of these cases presented in the U.S.A. with heat stroke), or DOCA administration. Chloride secretion in sweat may be high in parents of some cases.

This abnormality can be detected using a weighed dry piece of filter paper applied to the skin over the scapula and sealed in a 5 cm. (2-in.)-square polythene window. Active sweating is induced, and when the paper is soaked in sweat, it is removed, weighed, and the sodium chloride content estimated.

Nail clippings can be used in place of the sweat test.

N.B.—Since babies with mucoviscidosis are more subject to heat stroke than normals, the production of maximal rates of sweating must be carefully induced. The complete enclosure of a baby's body (other than the head) in a bag for the collection of sweat is dangerous, unnecessary, and has already caused a fatality.

REFERENCES.—Di Sant' Agnese, P. A. (1956), *Amer. J. Med.*, **21**, 406; Antonelli, M., Balloti, G., and Annibaldi, L. (1969), *Arch. Dis. Childh.*, **44**, 218.

SODIUM IN URINE.—

Normal Output.—8–15 g./24 hr. (as sodium chloride). The daily urine output is normally equal to the dietary intake.

Normal adults can concentrate sodium in the urine to about $0 \cdot 33 \, N$. Infants do not have the same power of concentration and full-term normal babies from 7–14 days old have a sodium and chloride clearance of about 20 per cent of the adult value. Premature infants have an even poorer clearance. Therefore, it is easy to render an infant œdematous with intravenous saline.

The kidneys tend not to excrete sodium when the plasma sodium falls below 135 mEq./litre. Also when the glomerular filtrate decreases, the normal process of tubular sodium reabsorption removes most of the sodium from the urine.

Physiological.—

Increased Output.—

1. Increased sodium chloride intake.
2. Postmenstrual diuresis.

Decreased Output.—
1. Low sodium chloride intake.
2. Premenstrual sodium and water retention.

Pathological.—
Increased Output.—
1. Adrenal failure:—
    a. Primary (Addison's disease).
    b. Secondary to hypopituitarism.
There is diminished tubular sodium reabsorption because of adrenal cortical steroid deficiency. The urine volume is increased, with loss of the normal diurnal variation, and an increased sodium and chloride concentration.

2. Renal:—
    a. Salt-losing nephritis. DOCA, cortisone, and ACTH are all ineffective. Also there is an abnormally increased rate of formation of aldosterone.
    b. Mercurial diuretics. The renal tubular reabsorption of sodium is inhibited.
    c. Carbonic anhydrase inhibitor. This substance causes sodium reabsorption by the renal tubules to fall.
    d. Renal tubular acidosis (Lightwood type).
3. Water imbalance. Urine sodium excretion may be increased in water intoxication.
4. Cerebral œdema and head injury. "Salt wasting" may occur, especially following injury or irritation affecting the hypothalamic region.
5. In any form of alkalosis and other conditions in which the urine is alkaline, potassium and/or sodium bicarbonate is excreted in the urine.
6. With inappropriate antidiuretic hormone (ADH) secretion, urine sodium output is increased in the presence of reduced plasma sodium levels.

Decreased Output.—
1. Low sodium chloride diet with adequate water intake.
2. Excessive sodium loss, e.g., gastro-intestinal, with adequate water intake.
3. Post-operative. During the first 24–48 hours after operation, there is "stress syndrome" with increased adrenocortical steroid hormone production.
4. Cushing's syndrome.
5. Steroid hormone administration, especially DOCA. In both (4) and (5) the urine volume falls, with low sodium and raised potassium output.
6. Reduced glomerular filtration rate. There is normal sodium reabsorption by the renal tubule cells from a glomerular filtrate reduced in volume, e.g., congestive cardiac failure.

N.B.—Diabetes insipidus. On a normal diet and adequate fluid intake, the daily output in the excessively large volume of urine is normal. Obviously the urine sodium concentration is very low.

SUGAR. *See* GLUCOSE

SULPHÆMOGLOBINÆMIA

Each sulphæmoglobin molecule contains one S atom more than hæmoglobin. Cyanosis becomes clinically obvious when 3–5 g. per cent of the total hæmoglobin is in the form of sulphæmoglobin. The pigment has no respiratory function, does not alter the red-cell life-span, and remains unchanged in the cells until their dissolution.

Pathological.—

Increase.—

1. Antimony compounds.
2. Acetanilide medication.
3. Phenacetin medication.
4. Bromide ingestion.
5. Sulphonamide therapy.
6. Nitrate ingestion (e.g., impure well water).
7. Nitroglycerin poisoning.
8. Sulphur, sulphides, and thiosulphate.

It is possible that these substances cause damage to the red-cell enzymes, resulting in the intracellular formation of the pigment, or there may be an association with the formation of hydrogen sulphide in the bowel.

Only if the red cells are lysed does sulphæmoglobin appear in the plasma.

Sulphæmoglobin has only rarely been described in the urine. It is probable that any cause of methæmoglobinæmia will also cause sulphæmoglobin formation if sulphur or hydrogen sulphide is available.

REFERENCE.—Halawani, A., Shaker, M. H., Abdalla, A., and Saif, M. (1956), *Lancet*, **1**, 190.

TESTOSTERONE IN PLASMA

Physiological.—

Normal adult males—0·7 μg./100 ml.

Normal adult females—0·04 μg./100 ml.

In men most of the testosterone circulating in the blood is secreted by the testes. In women more than half the circulating testosterone results from conversion of plasma androstenedione.

One per cent of the circulating testosterone is excreted in the urine as testosterone glucuronide and testosterone sulphate.

The maternal plasma contains 114 ± 38 ng./100 ml. and this level is unrelated to the sex of the fœtus.

Pathological.—

Increase.—

1. Virilizing tumours in women.
2. XYY males.

Decrease.—

1. Klinefelter's syndrome.
2. Cryptorchidism.
3. Hypopituitarism.

In female simple hirsutism, ovarian production of testosterone can be demonstrated following 3000 units of HCG i.m. for 3 days, testosterone production falling following diethylstilboestrol 5 mg. b.d. for 3 days.

Adrenal testosterone production can be demonstrated by ACTH injection, production being suppressed by dexamethasone 0·5 mg. 6-hourly for 2 days.

TESTOSTERONE IN URINE

Normal Range.—
Adult males—70 μg./24 hr.
Adult females—6 μg./24 hr.

REFERENCES.—Finkelstein, M., Forchielli, E., and Dorfman, R. I. (1961), *J. clin. Endocrin.*, **21**, 98; Camacho, A. M., and Migeon, C. J. (1963), *Ibid.*, **23**, 301; Papanicolaou, A. D., Kirkham, K. E., and Loraine, J. A. (1968), *Lancet*, **2**, 608.

THYMOL TURBIDITY AND FLOCCULATION REACTIONS IN SERUM

Normal Range.—
1. Thymol turbidity: 0–4 units.
2. Thymol flocculation: 0–+.
   One unit is equivalent to the turbidity produced by 1 ml. of fluid, which contains 10 mg. of protein per 100 ml., to which is added 3 ml. of 3 per cent aqueous salicylsulphonic acid. This is derived from the original standard of Kunkel and Hoagland (1947).

REFERENCES.—Maclagan, N. F. (1944), *Brit. J. exp. Path.*, **25**, 234; Kunkel, H. G., and Hoagland, C. L. (1947), *J. clin. Invest.*, **26**, 1060; Yeoman, W. B. (1955), *J. clin. Path.*, **25**, 252.

Physiological.—
1. The serum thymol turbidity and flocculation are low in newborn infants.
2. The thymol turbidity reading increases after a fatty meal, due to the absorbed fat, but the flocculation is unaffected.

Pathological.—
Increase.—
1. Viral hepatitis. The test is more useful in assessing the rate of recovery, although it may be increased early in the disease. It remains positive in convalescence after the cephalin cholesterol reaction has become normal.
2. Cirrhosis of the liver. *But* the tests may be normal in both portal and biliary cirrhosis. Possibly the bile-cholesterol-phospholipid combination has a stabilizing effect on the serum proteins.
3. Other diseases in which there is a rise in gamma globulin:—
   a. Lupus erythematosus.
   b. Multiple myelomatosis (both beta- and gamma-types).
   c. Sarcoidosis.
   d. Tuberculosis.
   e. Subacute bacterial endocarditis.

N.B.—It has been suggested that the serum thymol turbidity depends on the gamma-globulin fraction, and that possibly abnormal lipid protein complexes, and beta- or alpha-globulin fractions may increase the turbidity.

Normal serum albumin stabilizes the protein complex, and therefore, the higher the relative albumin concentration, the lower will be the serum thymol turbidity.

The serum albumin present in cases of viral hepatitis does not give this "protection", and hence the test is positive in the early stages of the disease.

THYROTROPIN IN PLASMA (TSH)

This glycoprotein, with a molecular weight of 26,000–30,000, secreted by the anterior lobe of the pituitary gland, acts on the thyroid gland by increasing iodine uptake and incorporation, stimulating colloid breakdown with release of thyroxine and tri-iodothyronine, and by causing cellular hyperplasia and hypertrophy of the gland.

Physiological.—

Very high levels occur within half an hour of birth, falling progressively during the next 48 hours, whilst the serum protein-bound iodine slowly rises.

Normal Results.—In euthyroid subjects of both sexes, above the age of 1 year = 1·8–10 μU./ml. The level rises following exposure to cold.

Pathological.—

Increase.—Hypothyroidism, with increased half-life.

Decrease.—

1. Hyperthyroidism (normal results may be obtained).
2. Hypopituitarism.
3. Following treatment with thyroid hormone preparations.

This is not yet a useful clinical test, although serum thyroxine response to i.m. TSH may become a useful test, since the patient receives no ionizing radiation and serum samples can be sent to a reference laboratory.

References.—Odell, W. D., Vanslager, L., and Bates, R. (1968), *Radioisotopes in Medicine—In vitro Studies* (Ed. Hayes, R. L., Goswitz, F. A., and Murphy, B. E. P.), U.S. Atomic Energy Commission, Series No. 13; Williams, E. S., Ekins, R. P., and Ellis, S. M. (1969), *Brit. med. J.*, **4**, 336.

FREE THYROXINE INDEX IN SERUM

The free thyroxine in the serum is directly proportional to the level of protein-bound thyroxine and inversely proportional to the free binding sites on thyroxine-binding globulin. The advantages in using the estimation of the free thyroxine index are:—

1. Increase in distinction of both hypothyroidism and hyperthyroidism from euthyroidism.

2. In normal pregnancy and during treatment with contraceptive pills thyroxine-binding globulin concentration increases in the serum, but in euthyroid cases the free thyroxine index remains normal. In these cases the serum protein-bound iodine concentration may be increased above normal in the absence of hyperthyroidism.

3. Serum thyroxine-binding globulin levels decrease abnormally in nephrotics, long-standing debility, uræmia, and in patients treated with androgens or corticosteroids, but in

uthyroid cases the free thyroxine index remains normal, even hough the serum protein-bound iodine concentrations may be bnormally low.

4. Estimation of the index can be used during replacement herapy with thyroid extract, to assess whether the correct lose is being given.

THYROXINE IODINE IN SERUM

Normal Range.—3·5–8·0 μg./100 ml.

Pathological.—
  Increase.—Hyperthyroidism. Serum thyroxine iodine rises above 7·5 μg./100 ml.
  Decrease.—Hypothyroidism. Serum thyroxine iodine falls below 4·0 μg./100 ml.

TOLBUTAMIDE TEST

After a diet unrestricted in carbohydrates for at least 3 days, and after overnight fast, 1 g. (or 30 mg./kg. body-weight) is injected intravenously in 10 ml. of fluid in 2 minutes. Blood-sugar samples are taken before injection, at 30, 45, 60, 120, and 180 minutes subsequently.

Normal.—Blood-sugar falls to not less than 30 mg./100 ml. at 30 minutes, and rises to about 55 mg./100 ml. by 180 minutes (i.e., at least 70 per cent of fasting level).
  Normal curves are found in:—
    1. Functional or reactive hyperinsulinism.
    2. Adrenal insufficiency. (A low curve may be obtained.)

Pathological.—
  1. Diabetes mellitus. Gradual slow fall in blood-glucose, with less than 20 per cent decrease in initial blood-glucose value. In diabetics with no available endogenous insulin, there is no response.
  2. Pancreatic islet-cell tumour. The blood-sugar level falls lower than normal, and remains depressed.
  3. Severe liver disease. Low curve.
  4. Acute pancreatitis. Response to tolbutamide resembles diabetes mellitus.
  5. Malnutrition.
  6. Azotæmia.
  7. Idiopathic hypoglycæmia in children.
The test is probably most useful in differentiating between possible pancreatic tumour and functional hypoglycæmia. It is important to have adrenaline and intravenous glucose solution available in case severe hypoglycæmia develops.

REFERENCES.—Marrack, D., Rose, F. C., and Marks, V. (1961), *Proc. R. Soc. Med.*, 54, 749; Marks, V., and Rose, F. C. (1965), *Hypoglycæmia*. Oxford: Blackwell.

TRANSAMINASE. *See* Alanine Aminotransferase *and* Aspartate Aminotransferase

TRIGLYCERIDES IN PLASMA

Approximately 100 g. of exogenous triglycerides are absorbed from the diet each day. In the serum chylomicra account for

10–15 per cent of the total serum triglyceride. (Only 0·5–1·7 mg. per cent is present as free glycerol, and 7·7–17·9 mg. per cent is present as glyceride-glycerol.) Normal values differ between the sexes and with age.

Normal Range (mg./100 ml.).—

Age	Male	Female
Under 25	77·7±16·9	75·8±30·6
25–34	83·3±26·4	73·0±22·9
35–44	96·6±21·2	88·6±27·0
45–54	101·0±36·0	84·7±26·0
Over 55	109·0±27·7	89·9±27·3
Overall	93·4±28·5	81·9±27·2
	(47–210)	(36–185)

Physiological.—Normal rise to peak values by 6 hours after a fatty meal. Normally low values are found in South African Bushmen.

Pathological.—

Increase.—

1. Diabetes mellitus.
2. Nephrotic syndrome.
3. Non-nephrotic uræmia.
4. Pancreatitis.
5. Following severe myocardial infarction.
6. Long-term oral contraceptives.
7. Zieve's syndrome.
8. Glycogen storage disease Types I and VI.
9. Essential hyperlipidæmia, Types I, III, IV, and V (Fredrickson classification).

Decrease.—

1. A-α-lipoproteinæmia (Tangier disease).
2. A-β-lipoproteinæmia (Bassen-Kornzweig syndrome).
3. Familial plasma lecithin : cholesterol acyltransferase deficiency.

REFERENCES.—Carlson, L. A., and Wadstrom, L. B. (1959), *Clin. chim. Acta*, **4**, 197; Lofland, H. B. (1964), *Analyt. Biochem.*, **9**, 393; Bagdade, J. D., Porte, D., jun., and Bierman, E. L. (1968), *New Engl. J, Med.*, **279**, 181; Boyns, D. R., Crossley, J. N., Abrams, M. E., Jarrett, R. J., and Keen, H. (1969), *Brit. med. J.*, **1**, 595; Gupta, D. K., Young, R., Jewitt, D. E., Hartog, M., and Opie, L. H. (1969), *Lancet*, **2**, 1209; Wynn, V., and Doar, J. W. H. (1969), *Ibid.*, **2**, 756.

TRYPSIN IN FÆCES

There is a very wide normal range of fæcal trypsin content in the adult.

In a child under 2 years of age, if a 1 in 50 dilution of fresh fæces fails to digest gelatin, it can be regarded as presumptive evidence of pancreatic fibrosis.

REFERENCE.—Harrison, G. A. (1957), *Chemical Methods in Clinical Medicine*, 4th ed. London : Churchill.

TRYPTOPHAN TOLERANCE TEST

Ten g. DL-tryptophan orally normally results in less than 50 mg. xanthenuric acid in the subsequent 24-hours' urine.

Pathological.—

1. In pyridoxine deficiency (vitamin B_6) the urine output rises to 120 mg./24 hr.

2. Urine indoles increased.—
    a. Hartnup disease.
    b. "Blue diaper" syndrome.
    c. Tryptophanuria (with increased tryptophan).
3. Kynureninase deficiency—excess xanthurenic acid.

REFERENCE.—Gehrmann, G. (1959), *Dtsch. med. Wschr.*, **84**, 1165.

UREA

UREA IN BLOOD.—
Normal Range.—
    1. 1 week old: 8–25 mg./100 ml. (1·3–4·2 mmol./litre).
    2. Adult:
        Males.—Mean=31·8±6·5 mg./100 ml. (5·3±1·1 mmol./litre).
        Females.—Mean=28·7±7·1 mg./100 ml. (4·8±1·7 mmol./litre).

Physiological.—
Increase.—The blood-urea rises in normal people on increasing the protein content of the diet. There is an increase with age, e.g., at 18–24 years, mean=27 mg./100 ml. (4·5 mmol./litre), at 55–65 years, mean=33 mg./100 ml. (5·5 mmol./litre).

$$\left(\frac{mg./litre}{60} = mmol./litre. \right)$$

REFERENCES.—Addis, T., Barrett, E., Poo, L. J., and Yuen, D. W. (1947), *J. clin. Invest.*, **26**, 869; Waters, W. E., Greene, W. J. W., and Keyser, J. W. (1968), *Postgrad. med. J.*, **43**, 695; Flynn, F. V. (1969), *Ann. Clin. Biochem.*, **6**, 1.

Decrease.—
    1. The blood-urea concentration is lower in the growing infant than in the adult.
    2. During normal pregnancy the mother's blood-urea is low.
        It is probable that in these two cases the amino-acid nitrogen is immediately reconstituted into new protein, and is therefore not treated as a waste product.
    3. Normal person on low protein, high carbohydrate diet. This is the basis of conservative treatment of anuria.

Pathological.—
Increase.—
    1. *Excessive Formation.*—
        a. High protein diet.
        b. Excessive body protein catabolism, e.g., fever, sepsis.
    2. *Faulty Excretion.*—
        a. Pre-renal Failure.—A low renal blood-supply leads to reduced glomerular filtration, e.g., as in congestive cardiac failure.
        b. Renal Failure.—Damage to the nephrons leads to faulty urine formation and excretion, e.g., nephritis, pyelonephritis, etc. The blood-urea begins to rise when the equivalent of one kidney is lost, or when the glomerular filtration rate falls below 10 ml./min.

N.B.—In the absence of pre- and post-renal failure, the blood-urea only rises after extensive damage has occurred, i.e., less than 800,000 intact nephrons remaining. Obviously the rate of development of damage will be important, since slowly developing damage will allow some compensation to occur.

    c. Post-renal Failure.—E.g., urinary tract obstructions.

Decrease.—

    Very low blood-urea levels may be found following transfusion of glucose solutions. The effect is a mixture of simple dilution of body fluids, protein catabolism reduction, and encouragement of diuresis. In the cases reported there was no evidence of either renal or liver damage. Prognosis was good.

    After hæmodialysis more urea is removed from extracellular fluid than from intracellular fluid, which results in:—

        a. Tendency to cerebral œdema, which resolves when dialysis is stopped.

        b. Unexpectedly rapid rise in blood-urea in the days immediately after dialysis is stopped.

REFERENCES.—Kark, R. M., Pollak, V. E., Soothill, J. F., Pirani, C. L., and Muehreke, R. C. (1957), *Arch. intern. Med.*, **99**, 176; Editorial (1962), *Lancet*, **1**, 845; Shackman, R., Chisholm, G. D., Holden, A. J., and Piggott, R. W. (1962), *Brit. med. J.*, **2**, 355.

BLOOD-UREA CLEARANCE.

—On a normal diet approximately 50–60 g. of urea are filtered by the glomeruli, and 25–35 g. of urea appear in the urine each 24 hours. From 40 to 50 per cent of the filtered urea is reabsorbed by passive diffusion from the tubules back into the blood-stream.

There is a direct relationship between:—

    1. Dietary protein and blood-urea concentration.

    2. Dietary protein and urine-urea concentration.

Thus, when the blood-urea falls within the normal range, the blood-urea clearance reflects the dietary protein intake, and when the blood-urea is raised to abnormal values, the blood-urea clearance reflects this abnormality also.

The blood-urea clearance is calculated in the same way as the glomerular filtration rate:—

$$\frac{\text{Clearance}}{\text{(Maximum)}} = \frac{\text{Minute excretion of urea in urine (mg./min.)}}{\text{Blood-urea concentration (mg./ml.)}}$$

$$= \frac{UV}{B} \quad \text{when the urine flow is greater than 2 ml./min.}$$

When the urine flow is less than 2 ml./min.:—

$$\frac{\text{Clearance}}{\text{(Standard)}} = \frac{U\sqrt{V}}{B}$$

$$B = \text{Blood-urea (mg./ml.).}$$
$$V = \text{Urine flow (ml./min.).}$$
$$U = \text{Urine-urea (mg./ml.).}$$

Normal Values.—

    1. Average Standard Clearance: 54 ml./min. (Range: 41–65 ml./min.)

    2. Average Maximum Clearance: 75 ml./min. (Range: 64–99 ml./min.)

The blood-urea clearance represents approximately 60 per cent of the glomerular filtration rate. Some authorities recommend correction for the body surface area, especially in children.

REFERENCES.—Moller, E., McIntosh, J. F., and Van Slyke, D. D. (1928), *J. clin. Invest.*, **6**, 427; Smith, H. F. (1949), *J. clin. Path.*, **2**, 266; Eastham, R. D. (1957), *Brit. J. Urol.*, **29**, 175.

UREA IN URINE.—

Normal Output.—10–35 g./24 hr. The output is proportional to the protein content of the diet, and also to the rate of body-tissue breakdown.

Forty per cent of the total urea filtered by the glomeruli is reabsorbed passively via the renal tubules back into the blood-stream. Very approximately, the rate of reabsorption is inversely proportional to the rate of urine flow.

Increase (negative nitrogen balance).—
1. Increased dietary protein.
2. Administration of 11-oxysteroids.
3. Excess thyroid action:—
    a. Excess thyroxine administration.
    b. Hyperthyroidism.
4. Post-operative state.

Decrease (positive nitrogen balance).—
1. *Normal.—*
    a. Normal growth in infants and children.
    b. Normal pregnant women.
    c. High carbohydrate low protein diet.

2. *Pathological.—*
    a. Convalescence (especially after a wasting disease).
    b. Liver disease, with reduced formation of urea.
    c. Toxæmia of pregnancy. Possibly a decreased rate of urea formation.
    d. Administration of growth hormone ⎫ Increased
    e. Administration of testosterone ⎬ protein
    f. Administration of insulin ⎭ anabolism.
    g. Renal damage (while the blood-urea is rising):—
        i. Nephritis.
        ii. Eclampsia.
        iii. Accidental placental hæmorrhage.
        iv. Renal metallic poisons, e.g., mercuric chloride.
        v. Incompatible blood transfusion, i.e., there is gross glomerular and/or tubular damage in the kidneys, leading to:—
            α. Inability to secrete any urine at all (anuria).
            β. Ability to secrete a small volume of urine only (oliguria).
            γ. Ability to secrete apparently normal volumes of urine, but unable to concentrate urine. The finding of a urine urea concentration of less than 0·5 g./100 ml., when the blood-urea is greater than 100 mg./100 ml., indicates gross renal tubular damage.
            δ. By excreting a large volume of urine throughout the 24 hr. (loss of diurnal rhythm) with a

fixed specific gravity, the blood-urea can be prevented from rising. This is the stage of compensating polyuria.

URINE UREA CONCENTRATION TEST.—No fluids are taken for the previous 12 hours (i.e., from 6.0 p.m. to 6.0 a.m.). The bladder is then emptied, and 15 g. urea (suitably flavoured) in 100 ml. of water are administered.

Urine is collected hourly for 3 hours.

Result.—

Normal.—In at least one specimen the urine urea concentration will rise to more than 2·5 g./100 ml., unless the urea has acted as a diuretic agent and the urine flow is greater than 100 ml./hr.

Pathological.—In renal disease, a concentration of 2·5 g. urea/100 ml. urine is not attained.

This is not a sensitive test of renal function. The administered urea is diffused throughout the body fluid and is not completely excreted in less than 8 hours in a normal person.

URIC ACID

URIC ACID IN SERUM.—
Normal Range.—

Children 4–14 years, mean=4·0 mg./100 ml. Range=2·0–6·4 mg./100 ml. with no sex difference.

1. Normal serum uric acid: 1·5–4·5 mg./100 ml.

$$\left(\frac{\text{mg./litre}}{168} = \text{mmol./litre.}\right)$$

2. The normal serum uric acid ratio in women/men=0·85 (until after the menopause).

3. Serum uric acid in the normal newborn is raised for the first year.

Physiological.—The renal tubules normally reabsorb 90 per cent of the uric acid filtered by the glomeruli.

Approximately 17 per cent of orally administered uric acid is eliminated as urea in normal men.

There is a significant increase in serum uric acid after severe exercise.

After fasting, or a high fat diet, the serum uric acid rises.

The normal "body miscible pool" of uric acid=1000 mg.

The gouty "body miscible pool" of uric acid=30,000 mg.

Serum uric acid levels tend to be higher in Group-B subjects and lower in Group-AB subjects.

REFERENCE.—Acheson, R. M., and Florey, C. du V. (1969), *Lancet*, 2, 391.

Pathological.—

Increase.—

1. *Gout.*—The serum level may rise above 6·0 mg./100 ml. in men, or 5·5 mg./100 ml. in women. Possibly the rise is due to increased renal tubular reabsorption. 25 per cent of patients' relatives have raised serum-uric acid levels

also, but without symptoms of gout (possibly the effect of a single autosomal dominant gene).

2. *Gross Tissue Destruction* (i.e., increased nucleoprotein breakdown).—
   a. Pneumonia.
   b. Eclampsia (some cases).

3. *Excessive Nucleoprotein Turnover.*—
   a. Myeloid leukæmia.
   b. Myeloid dysplasia.
   c. Treatment of myeloid leukæmia with nitrogen mustards, myeleran, etc.
   d. Hæmolytic anæmia.
   e. Pernicious anæmia (especially after treatment).
   f. Primary and secondary polycythæmia.

4. *Renal Failure to excrete Uric Acid.*—Uræmia.

5. *Pyrazinamide Therapy.*—Treatment of pulmonary tuberculosis with pyrazinamide (1·5–3 g./24 hr.) causes the serum uric acid to rise to 6–9·5 mg./100 ml.

6. *Primary Hyperoxaluria.*

7. *Hypoparathyroidism.*

8. *Coronary Artery Disease.*

9. *Mongolism.* Some cases.

10. *Athetoid Cerebral Palsy* with mental deficiency and self-mutilation. This rare condition is found in males with serum uric acid levels of 11–13 mg./100 ml. ≈ Lesch–Nyham syndrome

11. *Heavy Chain (Protein) Disease.*

12. *Von Gierke's Glycogen Storage Disease.*

13. *Lead Poisoning* (moonshine whisky causing "saturnine gout").

14. *Excessive Ethyl Alcohol Intake.*

15. *Launois-Bensaude Adenolipomatosis.*

16. *Type III hyperlipoproteinæmia.*

17. *A-α-lipoproteinæmia (Tangier Disease).*

REFERENCE.—Hoefnagel, D. (1965), *J. ment. Defic. Res.*, **9**, 69.

Decrease.—

1. *Hepatolenticular Degeneration (Wilson's Disease).*— Renal tubular reabsorption of uric acid is reduced, possibly as a result of damage to the tubule cells by excess unbound copper.

2. *Fanconi Syndrome.*—There is possibly a congenital tubular defect resulting in decreased reabsorption.

3. *Acromegaly.*—Some cases.

4. *Insulin Injection.*—Temporary reduction only.

5. *Uricosuric Drugs.*—
   a. Atophan.
   b. Cinchophen.
   No → c. Allopurinol (isomer of hypoxanthine) inhibits xanthine oxidase.
   d. Dicoumarol.
   e. Ethyl biscoumacetate, etc.
   f. Cortisone.
   g. Probenecid.
   h. Phenylbutazone.
   i. Salicylates.

j. Sulphoxyphenylpyrazolidine.

k. Thiophenylpyrazolidine.

N.B.—Colchicine, while dramatically relieving an acute attack of gout, has no obvious effect on the serum-uric acid level. In true gout the serum level may often be found to be normal. Thus, the diagnosis is most frequently made on clinical signs and symptoms. Serial estimations in known cases are useful, following treatment with uricosuric drugs.

The various methods for estimation of serum uric acid do not give identical results. The specific uricase method is not in general use.

REFERENCES.—Aponté, G. E., and Fetter, T. R. (1954), *Amer. J. clin. Path.*, 24, 1363; Lous, P., and Sylvest, O. (1954), *Scand. J. clin. Lab. Invest.*, 6, 40; Maclachlan, M. J., and Rodnan, E. P. (1967), *Amer. J. Med.*, 42, 38; Harkness, R. A., and Nicol, A. D. (1969), *Arch. Dis. Childh.*, 44, 773.

URIC ACID IN URINE.—

Normal Output.—

1. On normal diet—0·2–0·5 g./24 hr.
2. On high purine diet—Up to 2 g./24 hr.

Source.—

1. Exogenous (purines in the diet).
2. Endogenous (tissue nucleoprotein metabolism). Up to 90 per cent of the uric acid filtered by the glomeruli is reabsorbed by the renal tubules.

Physiological.—

Increase.—High purine diet.

Decrease.—High carbohydrate, high fat, low protein diet.

Pathological.—

Increase.—

1. *Increased Nucleoprotein Catabolism.*—

   a. Leukæmia, especially chronic myeloid leukæmia. Following successful treatment with myleran, or mercaptopurines, there is a gross increase in urine uric acid output, coincident with the falling white blood-cell count.

   b. Polycythæmia vera.

   c. Treatment of spontaneous remission in pernicious anæmia.

   d. There may be a moderate increase in uric acid output during therapy with ACTH or cortisone.

   e. Radiotherapy of lymphosarcoma and lymphatic leukæmia.

   f. Launois-Bensaude adenolipomatosis.

2. *Decreased Renal Tubular Reabsorption.*—

   a. Uricosuric drugs. (*See* URIC ACID IN SERUM.)

   b. Hepatolenticular degeneration (Wilson's disease).

   c. Some cases after ACTH or cortisone.

Decrease.—Allopurinol. Increased xanthine and hypo-xanthine output, with grossly reduced uric acid output.

N.B.—The urine uric acid/creatinine ratio is not a useful index of adrenocortical activity. Estimation of urine uric acid is not often useful in clinical practice.

UROBILINOGEN

UROBILINOGEN IN URINE.—
Normal Output.—0–4 mg./24 hr. (Output increased in alkaline urine and reduced in acid urine.)
Pathological.—
Absent from Urine.—
  1. Complete biliary obstruction (with no associated biliary tract infection).
  2. Complete suppression of pigment by the liver, e.g., after the first few days in acute infective hepatitis.
Increased Amounts in the Urine.—
  1. Constipation. There is a slight increase, due to longer action of bacteria on bile-pigments in the stools, and greater reabsorption into the blood-stream.
  2. Excessive hæmolysis:—
      a. E.g., acholuric jaundice.
      b. Blood-transfusion reaction due to incompatible blood transfusion, if renal damage does not prevent urine flow.
  3. Post-hæmorrhage into tissues:—
      a. Pulmonary infarction.
      b. After severe bruises.
        Hæmolysis occurs in the damaged area, and blood-pigments are released, to be eventually eliminated as bile pigments.
  4. Hepatocellular damage (if the biliary excretion of urobilinogen is more impaired than hepatic bilirubin excretion).—
      i. *With Jaundice.—*
        α. Early hepatitis (usually the first 48 hours, but it may persist for 1–2 days longer in some cases).
        β. Hepatic necrosis.
        γ. Congestive cardiac failure with hepatic anoxia.
        δ. Toxic damage to the liver with drugs, etc.
      ii. *Without Jaundice.—*
        α. Portal cirrhosis.
        β. Congestive cardiac failure.
        γ. Acute severe infection.
        δ. Recovery phase of acute hepatitis.
  5. Biliary obstruction, with infection of the biliary tract. In cholangitis very high concentrations of urine urobilinogen are attained. Probably bacteria act in the proximal parts of the bile-ducts, on the bile-pigments.
  6. In cases of fever in general.
  7. Possibly in some cases of pernicious anæmia.
  8. Possibly in some cases of lead poisoning, as evidence of increased red-cell destruction.

REFERENCES.—Gray, C. H. (1953), *The Bile-pigments.* London: Methuen; Bourke, E., Milne, M. D., and Stokes, G. S. (1965), *Brit. med. J.*, **2**, 1510.

UROBILINOGEN IN FÆCES.—
Normal Output.—40–280 mg. of urobilinogen (stercobilinogen) per 24 hours. 7–8 g. hæmoglobin are broken down (and synthesized) each day. 200–370 mg. bilirubin are excreted in the bile

each 24 hours, and much of this latter pigment is converted to urobilinogen in the bowel by bacteria.

Physiological.—

*Decreased.—*In infants and children, levels up to a maximum of 3 mg./24 hr. are usual.

Pathological.—

Decrease.—

1. Antibiotics. Some antibiotics eliminate the bacteria responsible for the conversion of bilirubin to urobilinogen, e.g., aureomycin.
2. Severe liver disease. The excretion of bile may be reduced.
3. Complete obstruction of the biliary tract. When very high serum bilirubin levels are attained, a little bilirubin may diffuse into the bowel, resulting in the appearance of small quantities of urobilinogen in the stools. Otherwise no urobilinogen is detected.
4. Low rates of hæmoglobin turnover:—
    a. Inanition and cachexia.
    b. Chronic low-grade infection.
    c. Some anæmias, especially aplastic anæmia.

*Increase.—*Hæmolytic anæmia with normal liver function.

*N.B.—***The fæcal urobilinogen, when expressed as a percentage of the total circulating hæmoglobin, provides a rough measure of hæmoglobin breakdown** (Urobilin Mauserungs Index of Heilmeyer).

REFERENCES.—Schwartz, S., Sborov, V., and Watson, C. J. (1944), *Amer. J. clin. Path.*, **14**, 598; Gray, C. H. (1953), *The Bile-pigments*, 48. London: Methuen.

UROPEPSINOGEN IN URINE

This proteolytic enzyme is normally excreted in the urine. There is a wide range of normal values: 10–40 units/hr. (milk coagulation method), with great variation from day to day.

Normal Output.—

1. Normal individuals.
2. Iron-deficiency anæmia, with normal hydrochloric acid content in the gastric juice.

Pathological.—

Increase.—

1. Stress (adrenocortical activity).

*N.B.—*One complication of continued steroid therapy is peptic ulceration.

2. Post-operative (adrenocortical activity).
3. After burns (adrenocortical activity).
4. Cortisone and ACTH administration both increase the urine output of uropepsinogen threefold.
5. Normal pregnancy. Moderate increase in output.
6. Duodenal ulcer.

Decrease.—

1. Pernicious anæmia, with achlorhydria.
2. Iron-deficiency anæmia with achlorhydria.

3. Post-total gastrectomy.
4. Gastritis.

REFERENCE.—Hill, A. B. (1954), *Lancet*, **2**, 1125.

VASOPRESSIN IN PLASMA

This estimation is not yet available.

VITAMINS

VITAMIN A IN BLOOD.—
Normal Serum Concentration.—100–300 i.u./100 ml.
One International Unit (i.u.)=0·6 μg. of pure beta-carotene=
0·3 μg. of pure vitamin A (since beta-carotene has 50 per cent
of the activity of pure vitamin A).

Pathological.—
Increase.—
1. Toxic signs and symptoms, with very high blood levels
have been reported in Eskimoes following ingestion of
excessive amounts of raw animal livers.
2. Idiopathic hypercalcæmia in infants.

N.B.—The total carotenoids (including vitamin A) increase
in the blood in:—

1. Chronic nephritis.
2. Nephrosis.
Decrease.—
There is no deficiency if the blood level is more than
20 μg./100 ml. Below 10 μg./100 ml., night vision is
impaired.

1. *Faulty Fat Absorption.*—
   a. Steatorrhœa:
      α. Sprue.
      β. Idiopathic steatorrhœa.
      γ. Cœliac disease.
      δ. Whipple's disease.
      ϵ. Intestinal diseases.
   b. Obstructive jaundice (the blood level may be normal in
   some cases).
   c. Chronic pancreatitis (some cases).
   d. Excess liquid paraffin intake.

2. *Liver Disease.*—
   a. Cirrhosis.
   b. Acute hepatitis.

REFERENCE.—Kaser, M., and Stekol, J. A. (1943), *J. Lab. clin. Med.*,
28, 904.

VITAMIN A TOLERANCE TEST.—After oral vitamin A:—
Normal.—A rise in the blood level occurs within 4 hours.
Impaired Absorption.—
1. Steatorrhœa, etc. (*see* VITAMIN A IN BLOOD).
2. Tuberculosis and other chronic infections.
3. Hepatocellular disease.
4. Malnutrition.
5. Cretinism and hypothyroidism.

Steatorrhœa.—The rise in blood level occurs later, and the peak is much smaller than in the normal.

REFERENCE.—Ditlefsen, E. M. L., and Stöa, K. F. 1954), *Scand. J. clin. Lab. Invest.*, **6**, 210.

VITAMIN B₁ IN BLOOD.—

Normal Values.—

1. *Plasma.*—The free form of the vitamin, which is diffusible, is present at a concentration of about 1 $\mu g.$/100 ml.
2. *Red Blood-cells.*—The erythrocytes contain thiamine pyrophosphate, the active non-diffusible form, at a concentration of 6–12 $\mu g.$/100 ml.
3. *White Blood-cells.*—The leucocytes contain 30–60 $\mu g.$/100 ml. as thiamine pyrophosphate.

N.B.—**There is no simple method for the estimation of vitamin B₁.**

Pathological.—

Increase.—

1. Leukæmia. (The raised blood level is accounted for by the high leucocyte count.)
2. Polycythæmia vera. (The raised blood level is accounted for by the raised red-cell count.)
3. Hodgkin's disease. (Lymphadenoma.)
4. Some cases of carcinoma.

(The significance of (3) and (4) is not understood.)

Decrease.—

A blood level of less than 3 $\mu g.$/100 ml. suggests a vitamin B₁ deficiency. Probably the leucocyte content is a more useful index of deficiency (cf. vitamin C in blood).

In Vitamin B₁ Saturation Tests, abnormally large doses of thiamine are required to achieve saturation in the following conditions:—

1. True vitamin B₁ deficiency.
2. Thyrotoxicosis.
3. Diarrhœa (prolonged).
4. Congestive cardiac failure.
5. Some cases of diabetes mellitus.

N.B.—**The pyruvate metabolism test is a far better guide to the presence of vitamin B₁ deficiency.**

VITAMIN B₁ (THIAMINE) IN URINE.—

Normal Output.—More than 50 $\mu g.$/24 hr. The range on a normal diet is: 100–200 $\mu g.$/24 hr.

Probably if any vitamin B₁ is found in the urine, deficiency can be excluded. With normal renal function, vitamin B₁ is a non-threshold substance.

VITAMIN B₆ (PYRIDOXINE) IN URINE.—Pyridoxine

dependency may be detected following excessive retention of pyridoxine load as measured by urinary output of 4-pyridoxic acid.

REFERENCE.—Gentz, J., Hamefelt, H., Johansson, S., Lindstedt, S., Persson, B., and Zetterstrom, R. (1967), *Acta pædiat. scand.*, **56**, 17.

VITAMIN B₁₂ IN SERUM.—

Normal Range.—The normal serum level is greater than 100 $\mu\mu g.$/ml., with an average value of between 300 $\mu\mu g.$/ml. and 400 $\mu\mu g.$/ml. Normally the bulk of the vitamin is bound to the alpha-globulin fraction. After an injection of vitamin B_{12}, the excess is free in the plasma. Vitamin B_{12} has a direct effect on desoxyribonucleic acid (DNA) synthesis in the marrow red blood-cells in pernicious anæmia.

Pathological.—

Increase.—

1. *Liver Disease.—*
    a. Acute hepatitis. The blood level may be 3–8 times the normal concentration. Predominantly the free form is increased.
    b. Cirrhosis and chronic liver disease. The blood level may be 3–8 times the normal concentration. The increase is mainly in the alpha-globulin bound fraction.
    c. Hepatic coma. The blood level may increase to 30–40 times the normal level. The increase is mainly in the free form.

    In (1) *a*, *b*, and *c*, the urine excretion is increased by 10–30 times above the normal output, and is mainly in the free form.

    The increase is in the alpha-bound fraction in :—

2. *Chronic Myeloid Leukæmia.*
3. *Polycythæmia.*
4. *Non-leukæmic Leucocytosis.*

REFERENCE.—Jones, P. N., and Mills, E. H. (1956), *J. clin. Invest.*, **35**, 716.

VITAMIN C IN BLOOD.—

Normal Range.—

1. Normal plasma: 0·6–1·2 mg./100 ml.
2. Normal leucocytes: 26±2 mg./100 ml.

Almost any plasma concentration is compatible with good health. The plasma may be devoid of vitamin C in healthy people, since the vitamin is carried mainly by the leucocytes. A constant plasma vitamin-C level excludes a deficiency, although a level of less than 0·2 mg./100 ml. is suggestive of a deficiency. A leucocyte level of less than 20 mg./100 ml. is also suggestive of a deficiency. A negative vitamin-C balance is indicated by a falling plasma level. Rapid restoration of plasma levels following oral ascorbic acid suggests no gross deficiency.

Clinical response to treatment is a much more useful indication of previous deficiency.

N.B.—A common method of estimation using 2 : 4–dichlorophenolindophenol estimates ascorbic acid but not dehydroascorbic acid. Since dehydro-ascorbic acid is converted in the blood to ascorbic acid, then probably the estimation of ascorbic acid (rather than ascorbic acid plus dehydro-ascorbic acid) is satisfactory. Using 2 : 4–dinitrophenylhydrazine, ascorbic acid and dehydro-ascorbic acid are estimated, but so also is 2 : 3–diketogulonic acid, which has no antiscorbutic properties.

REFERENCES.—Roe, J. H., and Kuether, C. A. (1943), *J. biol. Chem.*, **147**, 399; Crandon, J. H., Landon, B., Mikal, S., Balmanno, J., Jefferson, M., and Mahoney, N. (1958), *New Engl. J. Med.*, **258**, 105.

VITAMIN C SATURATION TEST.—After 700 mg. ascorbic acid orally in the morning daily, a 2-hour specimen of urine

collected at 3.0 p.m. in a non-scorbutic subject should contain 50 mg. of ascorbic acid. In cases of vitamin-C deficiency, "saturation" is only attained after more than three days of daily dosage with 700 mg. of ascorbic acid.

N.B.—

1. Some apparently normal individuals never appear to become saturated as judged by this test.
2. There is no evidence that saturation with vitamin C is essential for health.
3. The various proposed saturation tests use different loading doses of ascorbic acid, and different results may be obtained by using differing methods of estimation.
4. The white blood-cell ascorbic acid content is a much better guide to the presence of ascorbic-acid deficiency. Unfortunately, the estimation needs special apparatus, and is time-consuming.
5. During the performance of the vitamin C saturation test, it is essential that the urine be collected into glacial acetic acid if reliable results are to be obtained.

VOLUME OF BLOOD

Normal Range.—

1. *Total Blood-volume.—*
   a. 72–100 ml./kg. body-weight.
   b. 2500–4000 ml./sq. m. body surface area.

   In the newborn, blood-volume=85 ml./kg. body-weight, whilst in premature infant blood-volume=108 ml./kg. body-weight (due to increased plasma volume). Normal adult levels reached after 2 months.
2. *Total Plasma Volume.—*
   a. 49–59 ml./kg. body-weight.
   b. 1400–2500 ml./sq. m. body surface area.

The *Interstitial Fluid Volume* is three times as great as the plasma volume, and protects the plasma volume from marked change following loss.

In anæmia (other than immediately after hæmorrhage) the normal blood-volume is maintained by a compensatory increase in the plasma volume.

Increase.—

1. *Normal Pregnancy.*—Both the red blood-cell and plasma compartments increase, the greater increase being in plasma volume. This results in the apparent anæmia in normal pregnancy (i.e., hæmoglobin remains *above* 10 g./100 ml.). The total blood-volume increases by up to 45 per cent maximal at the thirty-second week, while the total plasma volume increases by 25–55 per cent and the red-cell mass increases by 20–40 per cent.
2. Polycythæmia vera (red-cell mass increased).
3. Occasional cases of congestive cardiac failure.
4. Administration of excess saline solution, glucose solution, or water after pitressin, results in increased volume until diuresis occurs.

5. Administration of glucose solution during hypothermia. The body enzymes act much more slowly at lower body temperatures. Glucose acts as a relatively inert expander of the extracellular space, until the body temperature rises again towards normal.

6. Over-transfusion with blood, plasma, serum, or dextran.

Decrease.—

1. Hæmorrhage. The plasma volume is rapidly restored from the fluid reserve in the interstitial fluid space. Rapid increase in the plasma volume compensates for the loss of red-cell mass.

2. *Water and/or Electrolyte Deficiency.—*
   a. Starvation, and water deficiency.
   b. Persistent vomiting.
   c. Prolonged diarrhœa.
   d. Addison's disease.

3. The blood-volume is said to be reduced in myxœdema.

4. Chronic nutritional anæmia. Plasma volume constant, but red-cell volume falls with falling hæmoglobin level. Therefore hæmoglobin percentage is read too high when compared with total circulating hæmoglobin.

REFERENCE.—Tasker, P. W. G. (1959), *Lancet*, 1, 807.

VOLUME OF URINE

Normal Range of Output.—
1. 1 week old: 50–300 ml./24 hr.
2. 6 months old: 350–550 ml./24 hr.
3. 3 years old: 500–700 ml./24 hr.
4. 10 years old: 700–1400 ml./24 hr.
5. Adult: 800–2000 ml./24 hr.
   The daily urine solute=600–800 mOsmol./sq. m. body-surface area.

The normal glomerular filtration rate is about 120 ml./min. Following obligatory normal reabsorption of salts and glucose with water in the proximal renal tubules, the filtrate reaches the loops of Henle with the same osmotic pressure as the plasma, and at a rate of about 20 ml./min.

In the presence of dehydration or antidiuretic hormone activity, most of this water is reabsorbed by the distal renal tubules until the urine flow falls to about 0·5 ml./min. In the presence of a water load, the water reabsorption is reduced, and the final urine flow can approach 20 ml./min.

The minimal normal urine flow required to eliminate all the body's waste products without increased blood-levels is about 600 ml./24 hr. in an adult. Normal tolerance=800–8000 ml./sq. m./day.

Physiological.—
Increase.—
1. Excessive water intake.
2. Increased salt intake. (Excess water is required to eliminate the excess salt.)
3. High protein diet. (Excess urea to be eliminated.)

Decrease.—

1. Low water intake, with high carbohydrate diet, i.e., the body protein is not so rapidly broken down, as would occur in starvation.
2. Excessive exercise and sweating.

Pathological.—

Increase.—

1. Pathological polydipsia.
2. Diabetes insipidus (i.e., deficiency of antidiuretic hormone). After ingestion of 1000 ml. of 1 per cent sodium chloride the urine volume in normal subjects and in pathological polydipsia is below 25 per cent of the ingested fluid. In diabetes insipidus the excretion rate is unchanged.
3. Diabetes mellitus. As the urine sugar content rises, glucose acts as a diuretic, i.e., the renal tubules are reabsorbing glucose at their maximum rate and the excess glucose prevents further water reabsorption.
4. Addison's disease and adrenal insufficiency secondary to hypopituitarism, and adrenalectomy. Deficiency of adrenal cortical hormones results in relative inability of the renal tubules to reabsorb sodium (and hence, chloride and water) and relative inability to excrete potassium.
5. Compensated renal failure. In chronic nephritis the urine eventually becomes isosmotic with the plasma ultrafiltrate, and 2–3 litres of urine are passed daily to maintain approximately normal nitrogen and electrolyte balance. The normal urine day/night volume ratio is lost.
6. Recovery phase in acute renal tubule damage. Before the power to concentrate urine is regained, a gross polyuria frequently occurs for a few days during recovery.

Decrease.—

1. Dehydration.
2. Low blood-pressure. The resulting reduction in glomerular filtrate and normal reabsorption by the renal tubules causes a gross reduction in the urine-volume.
3. Pre-renal deviation of fluid:—
   a. Nephrotic œdema.
   b. Cirrhosis of the liver, with ascites and œdema.
   c. Congestive cardiac failure with œdema.
4. Kidney damage:—
   a. Acute nephritis.
   b. Acute tubular necrosis.
   c. Acute pyelonephritis.
   d. Terminal chronic nephritis.
5. Obstruction of the urinary tract.

N.B.—**A daily fluid intake/output chart should be made in all cases where water and/or electrolyte imbalance is being considered.**

REFERENCES.—Platt, R. (1952), *Brit. med. J.*, **1**, 1313, 1372; Grossman, J. (1957), *Arch. intern. Med.*, **99**, 93 (review of body-fluid regulation); Jadresic, A., and Maira, J. (1962), *Lancet*, **1**, 402.

WATER CONCENTRATION TEST
(URINE CONCENTRATION)

Normally 130 ml. of fluid/min. are filtered by the glomeruli. After obligatory water reabsorption in the proximal renal tubules, about 20 ml./min. reach the distal tubules. Up to 19·5 ml./min. can be reabsorbed by the distal tubules, resulting in a final urine flow of less than 0·5 ml./min.

TEST.—On the first day of the test all fluids are withheld from midday. At 11.0 p.m. the bladder is emptied. The bladder is emptied again at 6.0 a.m. on the next morning, and the specific gravity of the specimen is measured at or near 15° C. in a vessel wide enough for the urinometer to avoid contact with the glass sides (specific gravity beads can be used).

Corrections.—
1. *Temperature.*—Add 0·001 to the specific gravity for every 3° C. above 15° C. Subtract 0·001 from the specific gravity for every 3° C. below 15° C.
2. *Glucose.*—Subtract 0·001 for every 0·27 g./100 ml. of glucose present.
3. *Protein.*—Subtract 0·001 from the specific gravity for every 0·4 g. protein/100 ml. urine.

Results.—
Normal.—The urine specific gravity is greater than 1·025.
Less than 1·025 Specific Gravity.—
1. Some normal individuals may have to restrict their fluid intake for more than 24 hours before the urine specific gravity rises above 1·025.
2. In cirrhosis of the liver, and also steatorrhœa, the normal diurnal variation in urine flow is lost.
3. In diabetes insipidus there is a massive persistent polyuria, with the urine specific gravity remaining at 1·010 or less.
4. When functioning glomeruli number less than 800,000 the specific gravity of the urine becomes fixed at about 1·010.

   Five units of pitressin tannate injected subcutaneously have been used in place of fluid deprivation. Fluid deprivation is obviously dangerous in cases with renal failure and obligatory polyuria, poorly compensated renal damage, or extrarenal uræmia.
5. Pregnancy bacteriuria. The concentration defect increases as pregnancy progresses. The lower the urine osmolality, the more difficult is treatment, and the higher is the incidence of pyelonephritis.

REFERENCES.—Miles, B. E., Paton, A., and de Wardener, H. E. (1954), *Brit. med. J.*, **2**, 901; Wolf, A. V., and Pillay, V. K. G. (1969), *Amer. J. Med.*, **46**, 837.

WATER DEPRIVATION TEST

The patient should be on a "dry" diet for 24 hours (i.e., food but no fluids).

1. **Polyuria continues.—**
    a. True diabetes insipidus ⎫ Urine specific gravity
    b. Nephrogenic diabetes insipidus ⎬ remains below 1·010.
    c. Unbalanced diabetes mellitus. ⎭

N.B.—**The urine specific gravity in diabetes mellitus will be high because of the abnormally increased sugar content. Clinical evidence of the disease will be apparent.**

2. **Polyuria ceases and Urine Specific Gravity increases.—**
    a. Normal person with previous raised urine flow.
    b. Hysterical polydipsia and polyuria. The urine specific gravity rises to more than 1·020 and the urine-volume falls to normal, if water deprivation is complete.
    c. *Incomplete Diabetes Insipidus.*—The urine specific gravity may rise to 1·016.

Subsequent administration of pitressin will differentiate between **1.** *a*, which responds, and **1.** *b*, which does not respond.

WATER EXCRETION TEST (OR URINE DILUTION TEST)

In adrenal cortical insufficiency, diuretic function can be restored within $2\frac{1}{2}$ hours by 50 mg. oral cortisone acetate. Maximum diuresis occurs in 5 hours. The effect lasts for 12 hours, and ceases within 18–24 hours of the dose. It is specific for cortisone and hydrocortisone only.

TEST.—Before breakfast the bladder is emptied, and 20 ml./kg. body-weight of water is administered, to be drunk within a period of 30–45 minutes. The fluid volume is not critical. The patient then rests, and the urine is collected each hour for the next 4 hours.

Normal Result.—The urine specific gravity falls to 1·002 during the ensuing diuresis.

1. 50 per cent or more of the total volume ingested should be excreted during the first 2 hours.
2. 80 per cent or more of the total ingested volume should be excreted during the first 4 hours.
3. The maximum rate of urine flow will exceed 2–3 ml./min.
4. The normal range of excretion after 1 litre of fluid orally is 230–1113 ml. in the first 2 hours (mean=813 ml.). This was found in normal patients in the age-group 13–72 years. This response is too non-specific to be useful as a test of renal function.

Pathological.—Impaired diuresis:—
1. *Faulty Water Absorption* (e.g., malabsorption syndrome).— There is prolonged retention of water in the intestines, with subsequent absence of diuresis, and occurrence of nocturia.
2. *Faulty Water Distribution.—*
    a. Gross œdema.
    b. Gross ascites, as in cirrhosis of the liver.
    c. Gross obesity.
    d. Dehydration.

3. *Pre-renal Dysfunction.*—Congestive cardiac failure.

4. *Renal Dysfunction.*—Renal damage with reduction in the number of functioning nephrons (resulting in inability to offer diuretic response).

5. *Primary and Secondary Adrenal Insufficiency.*—The previous causes of impairment (1), (2), (3), and (4) can usually be excluded on clinical examination.

REFERENCE.—Lamdin, E. (1959), *Arch. int. Med.*, **103**, 644 (91 references).

SECOND PART OF TEST.—If the results obtained are less than normal, repeat the test on the following day, after 50 mg. cortisone acetate orally, given 4 hours before the water load. (In some cases 100 mg. cortisone acetate may be required.)

Food and unaccustomed or excessive cigarette-smoking interferes with the diuresis.

In primary or secondary adrenal insufficiency, after adequate cortisone dosage, the diuretic response becomes normal.

Patients with myxœdema show slight improvement following cortisone, but recover fully after thyroid extract.

N.B.—**If the plasma sodium level is low, even cortisone will not produce a normal water diuresis, and water intoxication may develop.**

REFERENCES.—Oleesky, S. (1953), *Lancet*, **1**, 769; Taylor, W. H. (1954), *Clin. Sci.*, **13**, 239; Carrasco, M., Jadresic, A., and Lopez, E. (1962), *Lancet*, **1**, 401.

WATER EXCRETION TEST OF KEPLER, POWER, AND ROBINSON

With safer and more direct tests of adrenal function available, this test should now be discontinued.

REFERENCE.—Kepler, E. J., Robinson, F. J., and Power, N. H. (1942), *J. Amer. med. Ass.*, **118**, 1404.

XYLOSE TOLERANCE TEST

After 25 g. D-xylose orally in water, normal plasma levels being over 32·5 mg./100 ml., peak blood-xylose levels are reached by 2 hours, and pre-ingestion blood levels are reached by 5 hours, but there is great individual variation in blood levels in normal subjects. Gastro-intestinal disturbance often follows this size of dose, and a 5-g. dose is preferred. Renal excretion of D-xylose is proportional to its plasma level at any given time, and appears to be independent of the rate of urine flow.

After 5 g. D-xylose orally in water, the urine collected in the following 2 hours contains 0·7–1·7 g. xylose; and in 5 hours contains 1·15–2·4 g. xylose, the ratio of the 2 hr./5 hr. specimens being 39–81 per cent in normal subjects.

D-Xylose is absorbed from the duodenum and upper jejunum. It is not affected by intestinal bacteria or enzymes, it is not normally present in the blood, and is not absorbed against a concentration gradient.

Normal Result.—
- *a.* Normal subjects.
- *b.* Steatorrhœa due to pancreatic disease.
- *c.* Simple malnutrition.
- *d.* Post-gastrectomy (most cases).
- *e.* Cirrhosis of liver.
- *f.* Regional ileitis.
- *g.* Enterocolitis.
- *h.* Specific successful treatment of cases with reduced urine xylose output (e.g., gluten-free diet in case of steatorrhœa due to gluten sensitivity).

Reduced Urine Output of Xylose.—
- *a.* Cœliac disease. Steatorrhœa associated with gluten sensitivity.
- *b.* Addisonian megaloblastic anæmia (some cases).
- *c.* Sprue.
- *d.* Renal disease (cf. raised blood-xylose curve instead of flat curve found in *a, b, c*). Since the test is greatly affected by reduction in the glomerular filtration rate, urine-xylose output may be low in normal old people.
- *e.* Parkinsonism.

This test probably detects upper jejunal malabsorption defects. Its results correlate with folic acid excretion tests, but not with either fæcal fat estimations or serum carotene levels. Unfortunately xylose causes gastro-intestinal upset in many patients.

REFERENCES.—Fowler, D., and Cooke, W. T. (1960), *Gut*, **1**, 67; Santini, R., Sheehy, T. W., and Martinez de Jesus, J. (1961), *Gastroenterol.*, **40**, 772; Chanarin, I., and Bennett, M. C. (1962), *Brit. med. J.*, **1**, 985.

ZINC SULPHATE TURBIDITY REACTION IN SERUM
Normal Range.— 2–8 units.
One Unit.—
1. One unit is equivalent to the turbidity produced by 1 ml. of fluid which contains 10 mg. of protein per 100 ml., to which is added 3 ml. of 3 per cent aqueous salicylsulphonic acid (Yeoman, 1955). This is derived from the original standard:—
2. Three ml. of solution containing 1·15 g. $BaCl_2.2H_2O$ per 100 ml. is made up to 100 ml. with 0·2 N H_2SO_4. This suspension turbidity is equivalent to 20 units (Kunkel, 1947).

Pathological.—
Increase.—
1. *Liver Disease.—*
   - *a.* Acute hepatitis.
   - *b.* Cirrhosis of the liver.
   - *c.* Biliary obstruction with liver damage.
2. *Development of Antibodies.—*
   - *a.* Acute infections, after the acute phase, and during convalescence.
   - *b.* Rheumatic fever. Increases as the antistreptolysin "O" titre rises.
   - *c.* Chronic tuberculosis.

3. *Other Diseases in which the Gamma-globulin rises.*—
   a. Rheumatoid arthritis.
   b. Other collagen diseases.
   c. Multiple myelomatosis.
   d. Sarcoidosis (in active phase).

Decrease.—
   1. Congenital agammaglobulinæmia.
   2. Acquired agammaglobulinæmia.
   3. Acquired hypogammaglobulinæmia.

N.B.—**Although the serum zinc sulphate turbidity is directly proportional to the gamma-globulin concentration, in cases where there is gross dysproteinæmia (low albumin, reversed albumin/globulin ratio, or hæmoconcentration) " protection " effects may occur within the serum buffer system. It is thus possible to obtain " normal " results in pathological states.**

REFERENCES.—Kunkel, H. G. (1947), *Proc. Soc. exp. Biol., N.Y.*, **66**, 217; Yeoman, W. B. (1955), *J. clin. Path.*, **8**, 252.

EXUDATE VERSUS TRANSUDATE

Although the findings are not always clear-cut, the following generalizations are a guide to the nature of abnormal fluids:—

	EXUDATE	TRANSUDATE
Protein content	More than 3 g./100 ml. Fibrinogen present (clots on standing)	Often less than 1 g./100 ml. May be up to 2 g./100 ml. No fibrinogen
Specific gravity	More than 1·018	Less than 1·015
Glucose	Low if bacteria present	As blood concentration
Chloride	Related to the protein content	Related to the protein content

ŒDEMA FLUID

1. Low protein (0·1–0·9 g. per cent).—
   Cardiac failure.
   Hypoproteinæmia.
   Venous disturbances.

2. High protein (1–5·0 g. per cent).—
   Paralysis.
   Malignancy.
   Surgery.
   Idiopathic lymphœdema.
   Burns (4–6 g. per cent).
   Allergy (4–6 g. per cent).

REFERENCE.—Taylor, G. W., Kinmonth, J. B., and Dangerfield, W. G. (1958), *Brit. med. J.*, **1**, 1159.

DIAGNOSTIC SPECIALIZED ENZYME ESTIMATIONS

In the following sections, various uncommon but serious clinical conditions are listed, with their corresponding diagnostic enzyme deficiencies which can be demonstrated in various biological materials if laboratory facilities are available. Many of these conditions cause mental retardation, and such diagnostic aids are important both in enabling early treatment in affected infants where treatment is possible, and in the detection of affected families.

REFERENCE.—*Clinical Pathology in Mental Retardation* (Ed. Eastham, R. D., and Jancar, J.) (1968). Bristol: Wright.

ENZYME ESTIMATIONS ON MATERIAL FROM LIVER BIOPSY.—

Enzyme Deficiency	Clinical Condition
A-form of N-acetyl-beta-glucosaminidase	Tay-Sach's disease (the deficiency is also detectable in amniotic fluid)
Amylo-1,6-glucosidase	Type III glycogen storage disease
Argininosuccinic acid synthetase	Citrullinuria
Argininosuccinic lyase	Argininosuccinic aciduria
Carbamyl phosphate synthetase	Hyperammonæmia
Cyclohydrolase	Cyclohydrolase deficiency
Cystathionase	Cystathioninuria
Cystathionine synthetase	Homocystinuria (can also be used to detect heterozygotes)
Formiminotransferase	Formiminotransferase deficiency
Fructose-1-phosphate aldolase	Hereditary fructose intolerance
Galactose-1-phosphate-uridyl transferase	Galactosæmia
Beta-galactosidase isoenzyme	Hunter's syndrome
Glycogen synthetase	Glycogen synthetase deficiency
Histidine-alpha-deaminase	Histidinæmia
Para-hydroxyphenylpyruvate oxidase	Tyrosinæmia
N^5-methyltetrahydrofolate transferase	N^5-methyltetrahydrofolate transferase deficiency
Ornithine transcarbamylase	Ornithine transcarbamylase deficiency
Phosphorylase	Type VIII glycogen storage disease (inactive phosphorylase)
Proline oxidase	Familial hyperprolinæmia, Type I
Propionyl CoA carboxylase	Propionic acidæmia
Delta pyrroline-5-carboxylic acid dehydrogenase	Familial hyperprolinæmia, Type II
Sarcosine dehydrogenase	Hypersarcosinæmia
Sulphite oxidase	Sulphite oxidase deficiency

ENZYME ESTIMATIONS ON LYSED ERYTHROCYTES.—

Enzyme Deficiency	*Clinical Condition*
Glucose-6-phosphate dehydrogenase	
Pyruvate kinase	
Hexokinase	Congenital non-spherocytic
2,3-Diphosphoglyceromutase	hæmolytic anæmia
Triose phosphate isomerase	
Glucose-6-phosphate isomerase	
Glutathione reductase	
Orotidylic pyrophosphorylase	Hereditary orotic aciduria
Orotidylic decarboxylase	
Hypoxanthine-guanine-phosphoribosyl transferase	Lesch-Nyhan hyperuricæmia
Cyclohydrolase	Cyclohydrolase deficiency
NAD-dependent methæmoglobin reductase	Familial methæmoglobinæmia
Transketolase	Vitamin-B₁ deficiency
Aspartate aminotransferase	Pyridoxine (vitamin-B₆) deficiency
Arginase	Arginase deficiency
Argininosuccinase	Argininosuccinicaciduria (both homozygotes and heterozygotes)

ENZYME ESTIMATIONS ON LYSED LEUCOCYTES.—

Enzyme Deficiency	*Clinical Condition*
Arylsulphatase A	Metachromatic leucodystrophy
Alpha-galactosidase	Fabry's disease
Beta-galactosidase	Generalized gangliosidosis
Beta-glucosidase	Gaucher's disease
Alpha-keto-iso-caproic decarboxylase	Maple syrup urine disease
Methylmalonyl-Co-A-isomerase	
Methylmalonic acid-degrading enzyme	Methylmalonic aciduria
Propionate oxidase	
Propionate oxidase	Ketotic hyperglycinæmia
Sphingomyelin-splitting enzyme	Niemann-Pick disease

ENZYME ESTIMATIONS ON MUSCLE BIOPSY MATERIAL.—

Enzyme Deficiency	*Clinical Condition*
Alpha-1,4-glucosidase	Type II glycogen-storage disease (in homozygotes and heterozygotes)

ENZYME ESTIMATIONS ON TISSUE CULTURES FROM SKIN BIOPSY MATERIAL.—

Enzyme Deficiency	*Clinical Condition*
Beta-galactosidase + iso-enzymes	Hunter's syndrome and Hurler's syndrome

ENZYME ESTIMATIONS ON SEMINAL FLUID.—

Enzyme Deficiency	*Clinical Condition*
A.A.D. glucosaminase	Aspartyl glucosaminase deficiency

INDEX